THE PROTEIN PACING DIET

THE SCIENTIFIC BREAKTHROUGH FOR BOOSTING METABOLISM, LOSING FAT AND GAINING LEAN MUSCLE

NICOLE STAWICKI, RDN

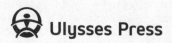 Ulysses Press

Published in the United States by:
ULYSSES PRESS
P.O. Box 3440
Berkeley, CA 94703
www.ulyssespress.com

ISBN: 978-1-61243-785-9
Library of Congress Control Number: 2018930774

Printed in Canada by Marquis Book Printing
10 9 8 7 6 5 4 3 2 1

Acquisitions editor: Bridget Thoreson
Managing editor: Claire Chun
Editor: Shayna Keyles
Proofreader: Renee Rutledge
Production: Caety Klingman
Front cover design: Hannah Rohrs
Indexer: Sayre Van Young

Distributed by Publishers Group West

NOTE TO READERS: This book has been written and published strictly for informational and educational purposes only. It is not intended to serve as medical advice or to be any form of medical treatment. You should always consult your physician before altering or changing any aspect of your medical treatment and/or undertaking a diet regimen, including the guidelines as described in this book. Do not stop or change any prescription medications without the guidance and advice of your physician. Any use of the information in this book is made on the reader's good judgment after consulting with his or her physician and is the reader's sole responsibility. This book is not intended to diagnose or treat any medical condition and is not a substitute for a physician.

This book is independently authored and published and no sponsorship or endorsement of this book by, and no affiliation with, any trademarked brands or other products mentioned within is claimed or suggested. All trademarks that appear in ingredient lists and elsewhere in this book belong to their respective owners and are used here for informational purposes only. The author and publisher encourage readers to patronize the quality brands mentioned and pictured in this book.

This book is dedicated to my sister Andrea and husband Todd for all their love and support, and to my dog Loco, for always standing guard while I was writing.

CONTENTS

APPENDIX 145

PART 1
THE RESEARCH

INTRODUCTION

Though there is a lot of information out there on nutrition and health, I still see clients who struggle to lose weight and end up yo-yo dieting for years. It's even harder for people who have desk jobs or are busy and cannot find time to exercise regularly. And no one wants to have to give up their favorite foods or spend hours cooking, especially if they already have very little free time.

I often hear that it is hard to know the "right" thing to do. It seems that every time you turn on the TV or computer, different nutrition and diet stories give different recommendations. How do we know the right thing to do if all the information is conflicting? When I was growing up, the fad was to stay away from fats and red meat and instead eat lots of processed, refined carbohydrates. I was taught that fat would lead to heart disease and weight gain. I remember eating margarine because we were told how bad butter was, only to find out down the road that margarine was actually loaded with trans fats, which are way more dangerous than the saturated fats in butter! My lunch as a teenager was often a bagel or cereal bars, which I thought were healthy because they were low in fat. However, they were made from processed, refined white flour and were almost entirely carbohydrates. All the "diet food" that was being sold was low fat and loaded with added sugars and chemicals. Even though America was eating low fat, people continued to gain weight.

It wasn't until I got to college that I really took a look at my diet and what the food I was eating was doing to me. This is what made me decide to major in dietetics and pursue this career. Not only did I want to eat better to improve my own health and well-being, but I wanted to help other people, as well. However, though I learned a lot about food and nutrition and really overhauled my diet, I frequently found myself getting nutrition information from less reputable sources. I still read nutrition tips from grocery store magazines because I hadn't learned that I needed to look at the source of the information. It wasn't until I became a dietetic intern and started to educate clients and patients that I realized how important it was to have an evidence-based practice. That is why this book is based on scientific studies that have proven to be successful.

Why Protein?

Many popular diet plans focus on increasing the amount of protein you are eating. Protein is so important in the diet because it has numerous roles in the body, and including protein foods at meals can help increase satiety, meaning you will feel full faster. Increased satiety alone can help with weight loss, because you will consume less total food during mealtimes. But while everyone can agree on the fact that protein intake is important, there are a lot of different factors to consider: How much protein is the right amount? When should you be eating it? Does it matter how much you exercise?

Over the past few years, a lot of studies have been done on protein pacing. The great thing is that the research was not done with people who were all the same; instead, the studies have focused on different groups of people with a variety of body types, fitness levels, and health goals. Protein pacing has consistently been shown to help people lose weight and reduce body fat, in addition to providing other health and fitness benefits. People have also found that protein pacing improved their athletic performance. By adopting a scientifically proven weight-loss plan like protein pacing, you are more likely to be successful in achieving your weight-loss, fat-loss, and health goals.

Using This Book

This book may include terms that are new to you, so I've included a glossary in the back to explain them. You'll see key terms commonly throughout the text, so it may be helpful to look at the glossary first.

The book is divided into two parts. Part 1 has a brief overview of why it is so important to have protein in our diets. It also discusses the different functions of protein in the body, why we need more protein when we are exercising, and some common myths about protein that I often hear when counseling clients.

Then, the science behind protein pacing is discussed in detail: the research, the results, and why it works. Using my insight as a Registered Dietitian Nutritionist (RDN), I will review the other health benefits of protein pacing aside from just losing weight, and offer guidance so that you can make protein pacing work for you. You will learn how to add the right type of protein to your diet and when you should be eating it.

In Part 2, you'll learn how to incorporate protein pacing into your life. You do not need to get out and start running marathons to make this work for you (unless you want to!). However, this book will address the types of exercise that you can do in addition to protein pacing to see results faster. I will also go over simple ways to add more activity to your day-to-day life.

Additionally, you'll find information on how to make easy changes to your current diet as well as food purchasing options and sample meal plans. I even share my own experience of testing a protein pacing diet, to give you an idea of what it might look like in your daily life, and to share practical results.

The book concludes with dozens of recipes to help jump-start the program and get you on your way to losing weight and reducing your overall body fat. Even if you aren't necessarily looking to lose weight, protein pacing can be an ideal plan to follow, as it provides many other health benefits and can help you achieve your fitness goals.

CHAPTER 1

WHY DO WE NEED PROTEIN?

The study of nutrition and how food affects our health and well-being has quickly become popular, though the science is still relatively new. Back when nutritional science first emerged, the focus was on dietary deficiencies and different diseases. For example, a deficiency in niacin, which is a vitamin, can lead to inflamed skin, diarrhea, and a change in mental status. Over time, food became more readily available and the focus of study changed. Nowadays, more research is being done on how nutrition and diet are linked to chronic illnesses, in addition to overall health and well-being. Some chronic conditions that have major nutritional components include diabetes, obesity, and heart disease.

To understand nutrition, it's important to learn about macronutrients. We need large amounts of macronutrients in our diets to support day-to-day activities and health. The three major macronutrients are carbohydrates, proteins, and fats.

Carbohydrates are the main fuel source for our bodies. After we eat carbohydrate foods, they are broken down into glucose, a type of sugar, which is then used for physical activity and to support different bodily functions. Glucose is the sole fuel source for our brains and red blood cells. Because of this, everyone needs to include carbohydrates in their diet. While carbohydrates are found in many healthy foods, such as potatoes, legumes, and fruits, they are also found in less healthy foods, such as soft drinks and candy. The type of carbohydrates we eat is extremely important. When choosing carbohydrate foods, it is best to choose foods that have been minimally processed and are low in added sugars. Sugars do naturally occur in some foods like fruit and dairy products, but foods high in added sugars should be limited, as they provide extra calories with minimal vitamins or minerals.

Fats also play an important role in providing energy to our bodies. When we are exercising, our bodies first use carbohydrates for energy, but after around 20 minutes, stored fat is used for fuel. Besides providing energy, fat has many other functions in promoting good health. We need fat in our diet, as it provides structure to cell membranes and insulation for nerve fibers in our brains. Fat also provides a cushion around some of our vital organs to help protect them (although having too much fat in this area can be dangerous, which I will explain in detail later). Another role of fat is keeping our skin healthy, as one of the most obvious signs of a deficiency is dry, rough, flaky skin.

Although dietary fats should be included in our diet, they are high in calories; if you consume too much fat, you will gain weight. You also must look at what type of fat you are consuming. Saturated fat is mainly found in animal foods, such as red meat and full-fat dairy products. Trans fats can occur naturally, but they are mainly produced when regular oils go through a process called partial hydrogenation. Both saturated fats and trans fats can increase your risk for heart disease.

Monounsaturated and polyunsaturated fats are mainly found in plant sources. You can identify them because the oils are liquid at room temperature. These types of fats are protective for your heart. Monounsaturated fats include olive oil, peanut oil, and avocados. Polyunsaturated fats include sunflower oil, walnuts, and flaxseeds.

The last macronutrient, which is the focus of this book, is protein. Humans need to eat some form of protein to survive and go about their day-to-day activities. Although it is easier to get complete proteins from animal products, vegetarian diets can provide adequate protein, as well.

Once protein is digested and broken down into its molecular components, called amino acids, it's used by every cell in the body. Amino acids are the building blocks of protein and are necessary to consume, since our bodies cannot produce them all. Until dietary protein is broken down into amino acids, it cannot be used by the body. One of the most important functions of amino acids is to help build and repair tissues in the body. And while most people know that protein helps build muscle, it builds a lot of other cells and tissues, as well. Amino acids support cell structure, repair worn-out parts of the cells, and create new cells. For example, red blood cells live for 100 to 120 days, and protein is necessary to help the body produce new ones. Protein is also extremely important in helping form antibodies, cells that are crucial to the immune system. Antibodies help us identify potentially harmful bacteria and viruses. Thereby, protein is necessary for us to have a functional immune system, which allows us to defend against many common microorganisms.

Proteins also have a job as messengers in our bodies, sending signals to other cells and organs to tell them to carry out certain functions. And amino acids help make up enzymes, which are used to carry out all the metabolic reactions that occur in the body; this includes both building reactions and reactions that lead to breaking down. All of these metabolic reactions are going on every minute of every day, and are necessary for our survival and basic functioning.

Lastly, proteins are used in our bodies for transportation and storage. They can be used to carry different molecules in the blood to various organs. For example, protein is an essential component of hemoglobin, the part of a red blood cell that carries oxygen in the bloodstream.

Protein as Fuel

We burn calories from all the foods we eat, but the effect is different for each food based on the thermic effect of food. The thermic effect of food refers to the increase in metabolism that happens after you eat a meal. Even though you consume calories when you eat, your body needs to use some of those calories to break down, absorb, and use the nutrients you have just eaten. Usually, we estimate that about 10 percent of the total calories we burn each day comes from digesting and absorbing the food that we eat.

The number of calories that we burn from our meals depends on the type of food that we are eating. It is much higher for protein foods than it is for carbohydrates or fats, meaning that we burn a greater percentage of calories trying to digest the protein foods.

The thermic effect of food is also different depending on the types of carbohydrates that you are eating. It takes more calories to digest and absorb complex carbohydrates than it does simple, refined carbohydrates.

Although sources differ on the number of calories we burn when digesting each of the macronutrients, we can estimate that we burn up to 5 percent of the calories when digesting fat, between 5 to 10 percent of the calories when digesting carbohydrates, and 20 to 30 percent of the calories when digesting protein foods. This is one reason why eating a higher amount of protein in our diet can lead to weight loss.

Protein Needs with Exercise

The amount of protein the body needs varies. If you are sick or have an injury, your body requires more protein to help heal itself. You also will need more protein if you are exercising or have a job that keeps you very active during the day. If you are exercising for prolonged periods of time, you have higher calorie needs, especially for protein. Without enough energy from carbohydrates and fats, the body must use the amino acids from protein for energy. If the amino acids are being used as an energy source for exercise, then they will not be available for other functions, such as muscle growth and repair. Thus, it is important to take in enough protein to guarantee your amino acids can perform their target functions.

It is common knowledge that you need to eat more protein when lifting weights. To build muscle and increase muscle size, you need to eat more protein than your body is breaking down and using. This is because participating in any type of strength or resistance training causes stress on the muscle. This type of stress will cause damage and small tears to the muscle. A special type of cell called a satellite cell is involved with muscle repair and building, but these cells cannot do their job unless you eat enough protein. You also need more protein when you do other forms of exercise, like aerobic exercise or cardio. When you are exercising, especially for a long amount of time, you can run out of glucose, which you usually use for energy. At this point, your body may start to use amino acids to help provide extra fuel so you have energy to continue the activity.

After exercising, you need to consume a protein-containing meal or snack so that your body can replenish itself. Without protein, your body would not be able to repair any muscle damage or increase muscle size. Even if you are lifting heavy weights, it would be very difficult to increase muscle size if you are not eating enough protein.

What Is Protein Pacing?

To put it simply, protein pacing means that you are spacing out your protein intake throughout the day. It is a type of program that can benefit many different groups of people, depending on their goals. The steady intake of protein has been shown to improve weight loss and fat loss, and protein pacing can be done without necessarily having to change your normal diet. Protein pacing has also shown proven benefits to strength and endurance, which would be helpful for anyone who is not looking to lose weight but just improve their overall fitness level.

Why Do We Need Protein?

Protein pacing is fairly easy to start. All you need to do is purchase a protein supplement that you will work into your daily routine, and possibly a shaker bottle or a special blender. You don't need to start any complicated meal preparations or start weighing out your food unless you want to, and you don't even have to start reading food labels (except for the protein powder label). That's pretty much it. Easy enough!

Protein pacing does not necessarily require a diet overhaul. This type of diet has been shown to help with weight loss and loss of body fat without participants having to change much about their normal diets. It can be a great way to jump-start your weight loss if you are not ready to make other dietary changes. Any other positive dietary changes you choose to make would just be an added benefit.

If you are making other dietary changes or cutting back on your calories, increasing your protein intake can help prevent you from feeling too hungry. Higher protein intake has been found to help improve satiety levels and keep you feeling fuller longer. It can be difficult to stick to any sort of diet or weight-loss plan if you feel hungry all the time, but that should not happen with this plan.

Taking in a higher percentage of calories from protein can increase metabolism through the thermic effect of food. It takes a lot more energy for your body to break down and process a protein food than it does a carbohydrate food or a fat. If you eat 2,000 calories one day and 30 percent of that is protein, and then the next day you eat 2,000 calories and only 10 percent is protein, you will have burned more calories from the first day even though the total amount of calories you ate is the same. Even if you are not changing your normal diet, you will be burning more calories just by increasing the percentage of calories you take in from protein.

The research on protein pacing and fitness measures shows that increasing total protein intake and evenly spacing it throughout the day, as well as participating in a varied exercise routine, can improve fitness markers. These improvements were seen in upper and lower body strength, as well as endurance, flexibility, and balance, as you'll learn about in the following chapters.

Protein pacing can be effective with either whey protein supplements or through whole food intake. It proved to be effective no matter what protein source the participant was consuming. This is important, because it means that there are more options for you if you'd like to start protein pacing. If you are the type of person who prefers to drink a supplement, then protein pacing will work for you. If you are the type of person who would rather eat whole foods, protein pacing will work for you as well.

Protein Myths

There are a lot of myths about protein, from how much you need to be eating to what is considered protein to what it can do for your health. It can be very confusing! A lot of the things you may hear seem to be contradictory advice. This section is meant to help clear up some of the most common protein myths that I hear.

You Need X Grams of Protein Each Day to Be Healthy

Despite what people will tell you, there is no set amount of protein that will work for everyone. How much protein you need is affected by a lot of different things. Someone who weighs 200 pounds does not need the same amount of protein as someone who weighs 150 pounds. Someone who does not work out does not need the same amount of protein as someone who is more active. Even people who exercise may need different types and amounts of protein depending on what type of activity they do. As I previously mentioned, your protein needs can change daily, especially if you are sick or have an injury. Just because someone else is eating 150 grams of protein each day does not mean that it is right for you to do so, or that you must do the same! The typical recommendation is that your protein intake should make up 10 to 35 percent of your total daily calories, but I will discuss this in more detail later in the book.

Eating a Lot of Protein Is Unhealthy

Eating a high-protein diet can be very healthy, depending on the type of foods you are eating. Animal-based proteins can be high in cholesterol and saturated fat, but there are a lot of animal-based proteins that you can include in a healthful diet. The role of saturated fat in heart disease remains controversial, so I wouldn't recommend eating a lot of proteins high in saturated fat until more research has been done on that topic.

If someone is eating bacon or sausage at breakfast, fast-food hamburger patties for lunch, and fried chicken wings with skin on them for dinner, then their diet would be unhealthy. They're getting lots of protein, but you can probably guess that the foods I just listed are high in sodium and overly processed. Of course, if these are your favorite foods, they can be eaten as an occasional treat. I am a huge proponent of the statement "all foods fit." However, there are plenty of other protein foods that are much better for you that you can eat regularly. White meat poultry, fish, and even lean red meat and eggs can be part of a healthful diet. Also, many of the protein supplements that you can buy have very little or no fat in them.

Your main dietary concern should be how much added sugars you are eating, not how much protein. Added sugars are problematic for several reasons. They are a source of empty calories that can lead to weight gain without providing any of the vitamins or minerals that our bodies need. Most Americans consume way more added sugar than is recommended. Research also shows that having more sugar in your diet increases the chance that you will develop heart disease, and that sugar may also have an inflammatory effect.

Throughout my years as a dietitian, I have regularly taught clients about cutting back on the amount of sugar they are eating, and most people are surprised about the amount of hidden sugar their diets have. In comparison, I have only told a handful of clients to cut back on their protein, and these cases have been related to their specific medical issues.

Protein Is Only Found in Meat Products

Most people, when they hear the word protein, will think of meat. While beef, chicken, fish, pork, and game meats are all excellent protein sources, protein exists in many other foods. Eggs and dairy products are also good sources of protein. You can also get quality protein from plant-based foods. Soy-based products such as tofu and tempeh contain a lot of protein, as do whole grains such as amaranth, quinoa, kamut, spelt, buckwheat, and barley.

For those who prefer to drink their protein, there are a number of companies producing high-quality protein powder, both from animal- and plant-based sources. You do not need to eat meat at every meal to get enough protein in your diet. However, plant-based protein sources contain less protein than meat products, so that is something to consider if you prefer plant-based protein sources.

All Protein Is the Same

There are a lot of things that can affect how healthful a protein food is and how much it will benefit your body. Some of the things that I look at when evaluating protein sources are the biological value, how processed the food is, the net protein utilization (NPU), and how quickly it is digested.

The biological value of a protein refers to how well the body is able to use the protein after it has been eaten. Protein foods that come from animal sources usually have a higher biological value than plant-based proteins. This is because plant-based proteins are usually missing at least one of the 20 essential amino acids. However, animal proteins can differ in biological value. For example, both whey protein and casein come from milk, but whey protein has a much higher biological value than casein. If you were debating between whey protein and casein based on biological value, whey protein would be a much better choice.

Another factor that affects protein quality is whether it has been processed. I frequently find myself telling clients to avoid processed meat products. I mean foods like bacon, hot dogs, and sausages—meats that have other ingredients added to them. This does not refer to items like ground beef or ground turkey, because even though they technically have been "processed," they do not have any other ingredients added. Processed meats have been linked to different diseases, like heart disease and cancer. They usually have a lot of sodium and chemicals added to them that do not naturally occur in meat products. Contrary to popular belief, red meat can be part of a healthy diet; it contains a lot of nutrients such as niacin, vitamin B6, vitamin B12, iron, selenium, and zinc. You do not get the same health benefits from hot dogs!

PROTEIN SUPPLEMENTS

Why are protein supplements so important to protein pacing? First off, protein supplements can be an excellent way to get high-quality protein into your diet, especially if you have little time for cooking. Consuming more calories from protein will increase how many calories you burn when digesting food, due to the thermic effect of food. Increasing your intake of high-quality protein can help you reach your health and fitness goals. Plus, drinking protein supplements, especially after exercising, can allow you to digest and absorb the protein more quickly, speeding up the availability of amino acids to your muscles. They are easy to purchase, and you can find high-quality protein supplements at many supermarkets and drug stores, in addition to finding them online. Protein supplements are an important part of many of the research studies that will be discussed in this book.

Net protein utilization is another factor that affects protein quality. After proteins are broken down into amino acids, they are used to varying degrees to build new proteins. The higher the percent of amino acids used, the greater the net protein utilization. Proteins with higher net utilization are more useful to the body and are considered to be higher quality. NPU is rated from 0 to 100. An egg, for example, has an NPU of 94, as does whey protein. While beans contain protein, they have a very low NPU, only around 39, although it varies based on the type of bean.

Lastly, digestion can vary between different types of protein. Some proteins are rapidly broken down and made available very quickly for our bodies to use, while others are broken down more slowly, providing more of a trickle of amino acids into our bloodstream. In Chapter 9, I will discuss how some of these factors actually can impact the benefits of protein pacing depending on the type of protein supplement used.

Switching to a High-Protein, Low-Carb Diet Will Help You Lose Weight and Keep It Off

The problem with high-protein, low-carbohydrate diets is that they are difficult to maintain for a long time. Many people think that they can follow this type of diet for a while, lose the weight that they want, and then go back to how they were eating before. And it's true that at first, this type of diet can help you lose weight. Eating more protein at meals will help you feel fuller for longer than you would if you ate a meal made up of more carbohydrates. This can help cut back on how many calories you eat. There is also some research that shows that levels of ghrelin (the hormone that affects your appetite) are lower after eating a high-protein meal versus a high-carbohydrate meal. Protein also takes longer to digest than carbohydrates, so just by including a small amount of protein in each meal, you should not feel hungry as quickly after you are done eating.

However, your body weight is still going to be affected by the total amount of calories you eat, so it is possible to follow a low-carb diet and not lose weight. Additionally, I have frequently seen that when people stop following this type of diet, they gain a lot of weight back once they start trying to include carbohydrates with their meals again. This regain of weight can be frustrating, and if they start a diet again, they can be constantly losing and regaining the same weight. This type of "yo-yo dieting" can have negative health consequences, so I always recommend making diet and lifestyle changes that are sustainable.

Eating a Lot of Protein Will Lead to Kidney Issues

Some worry that increasing how much protein they eat will result in kidney damage, which is not true. Our kidneys have a lot of important jobs, including filtering our blood, getting rid of waste products, and regulating the amount of water and electrolytes in our bodies. However, if you have healthy, normal kidneys, then you will not have an issue with this. While high-protein diets can be dehydrating, this won't be an issue if you are drinking enough water. I would be concerned about someone if they had pre-existing kidney issues, as they may need to watch their protein intake more closely. Anyone with pre-existing kidney problems should talk to their doctor about any special diet restrictions they may need to follow prior to changing their diet.

CHAPTER 2

THE PRISE STUDY: WHY PROTEIN PACING WORKS

I could not recommend protein pacing unless there was good, quality evidence that showed that it was successful. Fortunately, there is. Scientific research backs the idea that protein pacing, especially when combined with a varied exercise program, can help you lose weight. The great thing about the available research is that all the studies have been conducted among different groups of people with a variety of body types and different health and fitness goals.

One of the most notable studies on protein pacing, the PRISE study, was designed to look at the effects of protein pacing on overweight or obese people. The main researcher in this study, Dr. Paul Arciero, was involved in most of the studies that will be discussed through this book. PRISE stands for protein pacing, resistance exercise, intervals, stretching/yoga/Pilates, and endurance exercise, although not all participants were required to exercise. The study was noteworthy because it did not require any calorie restriction or dietary changes aside from the addition of a protein supplement, and it showed that people could lose weight just by adding a protein supplement to their diet.

The original PRISE study included a group of people who were either overweight or obese, and who did not participate in physical activity. All the people participating in the study were asked to consume a higher protein diet (up to 35 percent of their total daily calories). The research team was interested in seeing how spacing out protein intake throughout the day would affect protein synthesis, body weight, and body composition over about 16 weeks. Some of the participants were also assigned to different exercise groups to see if this would further improve their results.

The participants involved in the research did not have to change their normal diets, aside from ingesting the additional protein at specified times. There was no calorie restriction or calorie counting, no restrictions on any particular foods or food groups, and no complicated meal planning in this study design. This is important to note, as making a lot of dietary changes can be a huge roadblock to success.

In this study, participants were divided up into three groups:

Protein pacing. As you will see in many of the studies, protein supplements are very common in protein pacing. The first group of people in the study only took additional protein supplements. They were given three daily servings of whey protein. Each serving was equal to 20 grams of protein, providing each participant with an additional 60 grams of protein per day. The first serving was taken within one hour of waking up, the second serving was taken in the middle of the afternoon, and the third serving was taken within two hours of bedtime. Aside from the added protein dose, there were no other changes to the diets of the people in this group. There was also no additional required exercise.

Protein pacing and resistance exercise. The second group of people had to take the same type and amount of the whey protein supplement as the first group. However, this group also had an exercise requirement: They were required to participate in resistance training four times a week, with each session lasting about one hour. While the resistance exercise was meant to challenge everyone in the group, each person participating was given their own routine based on their individual fitness level. Participants in this group were required to take their afternoon dose of the whey protein supplement within 30 minutes of exercising.

PRISE. The third group of people in this study also had to drink the whey protein supplement (20 grams, three times daily), with the afternoon dose taken within 30 minutes of exercising. However, this group was required to perform a more varied exercise routine than the second group (this exercise was customized based on individual fitness levels, as well). They participated in a different type of exercise every day for four days each week, and each exercise session lasted 45 minutes to one hour. On one of the days, they performed resistance exercises similar to those done by the second group. On the other three days, the PRISE group participated in interval sprint exercises, cardio endurance training, and a combination routine of stretching, yoga, and Pilates. The cardio endurance exercises could have been anything as simple as walking, jogging, or swimming, to something more adventurous, such as rollerblading or cross-country skiing.

It is important to have numerous groups in a study to create a comparison. In this case, we can look at the results and see if the benefits came from protein pacing or if they came from starting an exercise routine. That is also why it was important that the participants in the study did not change their normal diet. For example, if the participants in the study had been asked to change their diets to something drastically different, we would not know if protein pacing was benefiting them, or if the results were from all the new diet changes. Even small changes that seem insignificant, like making sure each participant ate two servings of fruits or vegetables a day, could have affected the study outcome. If the fruits or vegetables replaced higher calorie snacks or increased fullness from the fiber content, it could have made a huge difference. By just having the groups start protein pacing without other dietary changes, the research team would know where the results were actually coming from.

PRISE Study Results

What were the results of the PRISE study, and why do they matter? I will go through all the measures that the researchers looked at and what the results showed for each group.

Weight loss and fat loss. All three groups saw weight loss, fat loss, and decreased total body fat, with or without exercise. This is interesting to me as a dietitian, as initially, I would not have thought that protein pacing alone would have led to weight loss, especially considering that the participants in this study were all overweight or obese with sedentary lifestyles.

Decrease in dangerous fat. All three groups ended up losing abdominal fat and visceral adipose tissue. Visceral adipose tissue, which is the type of fat in our abdomens and around our internal organs, is more dangerous than other types of body fat and is connected with many diseases. Even though any total fat loss would be a positive result, losing this type of fat will have more of an impact on your health overall.

The groups that did protein pacing with exercise saw the most significant loss of visceral adipose tissue. Although the protein pacing group did not lose a significant amount of visceral adipose tissue, any loss is desirable. And since all groups ended up losing abdominal fat and visceral adipose tissue, this also led to a decrease in waist circumference for the participants.

Most participants also saw a reduction in subcutaneous adipose tissue, which is the fat found under the skin. Having excess subcutaneous adipose tissue is safer than having excess visceral adipose tissue, as this type of fat is not linked with an increased disease risk. Interestingly, subcutaneous adipose tissue decreased in the protein pacing group and the PRISE group; however, the protein pacing plus resistance training group did not see any significant difference. Even though this type of fat is not as dangerous as visceral adipose tissue, loss of both types of fat is beneficial for anyone who is overweight or obese.

Increase in lean body mass. All the groups in this study had an increase in their total lean body mass percentage. Lean body mass refers to the total amount of weight that a person has that is not made up of fat. The changes were significant in the protein pacing plus resistance training group and the PRISE group. Considering that both groups were participating in activities that would increase muscle strength, it is not surprising that they would see the greatest increase in lean body mass. The total greatest increase in lean body mass was seen in the PRISE group, which is likely because these participants were doing a variety of different activities and challenging their muscles in a number of different ways. However, even without exercise, the group that was only taking whey supplements still saw an increase in lean body mass.

The lean body mass in the arms and legs of participants was measured before and after the study. Arm lean body mass increased in the protein pacing plus resistance training group and the PRISE group, but stayed the same in the group just doing protein pacing. Interestingly, the protein pacing group had a slight decrease in the amount of lean body mass in their legs, likely because they were not exercising, so there could have been some muscle loss along with fat loss. The amount stayed the same in the other two groups.

Improved insulin sensitivity. Insulin sensitivity was measured by testing fasting blood glucose levels and insulin levels. The people in the protein pacing plus resistance training group and the PRISE group had decreased glucose and insulin levels, meaning they had improved insulin sensitivity (or decreased insulin resistance). Even though the protein pacing group did not show much improvement in fasting blood glucose and insulin levels, weight loss and reduced body fat could slow down the development of insulin resistance in individuals at risk.

Additionally, those in the protein pacing plus resistance training group and the PRISE group had increases in adiponectin levels. The increase in adiponectin levels may relate to the improvement in insulin sensitivity in these two groups, since adiponectin is a protein that has a role in regulating how our bodies respond to insulin. Usually, we would see increases in adiponectin levels with exercise, which was the case in this study, as well.

Feelings of hunger and satiety. In the PRISE study, there was actually no change in the feelings of hunger and satiety among the participants in all three groups. At first, this seems very unexpected. Haven't we been told that if we eat more protein, we will feel less hungry? Many other research studies have shown that protein intake can affect hunger and satiety, so why not in this group? There actually may be a very simple explanation.

As I've discussed, the people in this study did not have to change their original diets. They were still eating all the same foods and in the same amounts. No one in this study had to restrict how many calories they were eating; they were told to follow their normal diet. This may be the reason that the participants did not feel less hungry. They might not have had any improvement in their hunger levels because they were not hungry to begin with. Had the people in this study been placed on a calorie-restricted diet, we may have seen more of an impact with the whey protein supplement on their hunger levels.

Takeaways

Based on this study, protein pacing, especially when combined with a well-rounded exercise program, demonstrated a lot of positive benefits. However, even if you are not exercising, the PRISE study shows that protein pacing alone will reduce waist circumference, total weight, and total body fat, including the more dangerous visceral adipose tissue. Reducing waist circumference and visceral adipose tissue is important for health and disease prevention, especially when it comes to heart disease and type 2 diabetes. No matter what, any type of weight loss can be beneficial if your BMI is above the normal range and you are already showing some of the risk factors for metabolic syndrome. While it can be more difficult for someone with insulin resistance to lose weight initially, overall weight loss can help reduce insulin resistance and improve blood sugar levels, so it is important for individuals with these conditions to try and lose weight before they develop serious health problems.

Significantly, the participants changed the total amount of protein they were eating. Prior to the start of the study, the average amount of protein eaten per participant was 18 to 19 percent of total calories consumed. After the participants starting protein pacing, the average amount of protein eaten among all three groups was 25 to 28 percent. This is well within the typical suggested protein range, which is 10 to 35 percent of calories consumed.

The change in how much protein was consumed was the reason why this study led to weight loss and fat loss, even though the participants were eating their normal number of calories. As discussed earlier, the thermic effect of food is much higher for protein foods than it is for carbohydrates and fats. Even without exercise, an increase in how much protein someone is eating would require more calories to be burned for digestion and absorption to occur. So, by eating a greater percentage of calories from protein, you would have a higher metabolic rate than if you ate a greater percentage of your calories from carbohydrates or fats. And even though there were more significant results for the groups in the PRISE study that added an exercise routine, protein pacing on its own produced positive results.

CHAPTER 3

WHEY PROTEIN VS. SOY PROTEIN

Protein supplements are an important part of protein pacing. When following a protein pacing diet, protein supplements provide high-quality protein with very little extra calories from carbohydrate and fat. Including protein supplements in your diet is the easiest way to start protein pacing, as it requires very little work or preparation. Whey protein has long been considered the best type of protein that you could buy. It is very popular in the bodybuilding community, and I personally know a lot of people who use whey protein to help meet their fitness goals. Now that I have researched it myself, I see why whey is the gold standard of protein.

If we are comparing whey protein to soy protein, the most obvious difference is the source. Whey protein is made from an animal source. When cheese is made from cow's milk, the liquid leftover byproduct is referred to as whey. The liquid whey is then treated so that the protein solids are removed from the liquid. When you are buying supplements, these protein solids are what is referred to as whey protein. On the other hand, soy protein is completely plant-based and comes from the soybean plant. Even though soy protein is plant-based, it is still considered a complete protein because it contains all the essential amino acids.

When looking at the amino acid content of both proteins, soy protein actually contains more glutamine than whey protein does. Glutamine is not normally an essential amino acid, but it becomes essential during times of metabolic stress, such as when someone suffers trauma or a burn. It is also very important for muscle growth and repair, and is often taken as a supplement on its own. However, taking a supplement that contains a single amino acid, such as glutamine, would not be necessary for the average person.

Aside from any potential digestive issues related to lactose (see sidebar, page 34), whey protein is digested and absorbed rather quickly. After drinking a whey protein supplement, amino acids from the whey can show up in the blood in as little as 15 to 20 minutes. This is one of the reasons why whey protein supplements are so popular after a workout. Due to the quick digestibility, they are ideal for muscle recovery. Soy is also very digestible and is favored by those who want to limit their intake of animal products. In comparison, the milk protein casein (page 91) takes a lot more work for the body to digest, so it takes much longer.

Earlier, it was discussed that different types of protein have different biological values. Biological value refers to how much of a protein can be used by the body, and how efficiently. If you compare whey protein to soy protein, our bodies are better at absorbing and using whey protein. Therefore, whey has a much higher biological value than soy does. Whey protein also has a higher net protein utilization than soy protein, meaning that more amino acids from the whey supplement would be used to build new protein. Overall, whey is a higher quality protein than soy.

Studying the Benefits of Whey vs. Soy Protein

Although the PRISE study reviewed in Chapter 2 clearly showed the benefits of protein pacing, I wanted to look at other studies on the topic to see if this type of diet would consistently produce the same results. A 2011 study published in the *Journal of Nutrition* compared the effects of whey and soy supplements when added to the normal diets of overweight and obese individuals. I was interested in this particular study to see if there would be a difference in the results produced by whey compared to soy, and if it would back up the PRISE study regarding the benefits of whey protein supplementation.

Like in the PRISE study, the groups of people in this study were not required to change their normal diets or restrict how many calories they were eating. They were also overweight or obese, with a BMI between 28 and 38. And, as in the PRISE study, the goal was to determine exactly what the results would be from taking an additional protein supplement daily, without making any other dietary changes that could have led to misleading results.

This study divided participants into three groups and lasted for three weeks. All participants were given one supplement packet twice a day (once in the morning with breakfast, and once in the evening with dinner). The first group took a whey protein supplement that had 27.5 grams of protein per packet; the second group took a soy protein supplement that had 28.1 grams of protein per packet; and the last group was the control group taking maltodextrin, which is a carbohydrate that is normally used as a food additive. All the supplements contained approximately 400 calories. Although there was a slight difference in the amount of protein between the whey and soy packets, it was not significant, as the difference was less than 2 grams per day.

Both the whey and soy protein groups consumed significantly more protein daily than those in the carbohydrate control group, although the daily calories among all the groups was very similar. Despite the similar doses of protein, I found the results very surprising.

Reduced body weight and total body fat. At the end of the study, the group that was drinking the whey protein supplement had lower total fat mass than the soy protein or carbohydrate group. The whey protein group also had lost weight over the course of the study, while the participants drinking the carbohydrate supplement had gained weight. Relatedly, waist circumference was lower in the people consuming whey protein than in the soy protein or carbohydrate group. This is something to consider in your protein supplement selection if you are looking to reduce abdominal fat, especially considering how this type of fat is related to potential health issues.

It should be noted that the soy protein group did not have a significant change in weight or waist circumference during this study. During the study, only the whey protein group had a significant change in their carbohydrate intake, which would explain why the soy protein group would not have had a significant weight reduction.

Appetite change. Like those in the PRISE study, the participants in this study did not see any differences in hunger, satiety, or feelings of fullness. This may also be because the participants did not have to change their normal diets, and were not calorically restricted, so they were not feeling hungry to begin with. Interestingly, though, people who consumed whey protein had lower ghrelin concentrations than those in the soy protein or carbohydrate group. Ghrelin is the hormone that helps regulate appetite by increasing hunger. So even though none of the participants reported changes in their hunger levels, the reduced ghrelin levels likely helped control the appetite of those in the whey protein group. Surprisingly, the soy protein group did not have reduced ghrelin levels. And though there were no significant differences in carbohydrate consumption among any of the groups at the beginning of the study, by the end of the treatment period, the people in the whey protein group were actually consuming fewer carbohydrates.

Takeaways

There are likely several factors that led to weight loss for the whey protein group. A big factor that likely contributed to weight loss is the thermic effect of food. Since the participants were taking in more protein than they were before, they would be burning more calories simply from the change in their intake, since protein requires more energy to be used for the body to break it down. Even though the whey protein group did not report changes in hunger or fullness, they had lower levels of ghrelin, the hunger hormone, so they were likely consuming less than they normally would have. The whey protein group also likely lost some weight because of decreased carbohydrate intake. They were not eating a low-carbohydrate diet by any means, but this was the only group that saw a change in carbohydrate intake.

One concern about consuming whey protein is that it is made of cow's milk. Anyone with a milk allergy needs to be careful to read supplement labels to make sure they are not eating something that can be dangerous to them. Most people who are allergic to milk are allergic to casein, which is a different protein than whey, but it is still something to be aware of. The other concern about whey protein is lactose intolerance. After processing, whey protein powder usually contains very little lactose, but there is always the possibility that some may be present. The amount of lactose left also depends on what type of whey protein you buy, which is further discussed on page 88. Anyone who is especially sensitive to lactose should try a small amount of whey protein powder to make sure it does not cause any digestive issues.

Now, it is possible that the change in carbohydrate intake is related to the change in ghrelin levels. For example, let's say someone is used to eating a lot of simple carbohydrate snacks. Simple carbohydrates are typically not filling, and it is easy to eat a lot of them, especially when it comes to snack foods. Once that person starts protein pacing, leading to reduced ghrelin levels, they might wind up eating fewer snacks, which is a possible reason for the change in carbohydrate intake. While it is impossible to know for sure why the whey protein group started eating fewer carbohydrates, this scenario is one potential reason.

For a more drastic weight loss, it may be necessary to make other dietary changes, but protein pacing with a whey protein supplement can easily be a starting point for someone who is not ready to make big changes yet. Unlike the PRISE study, none of the treatment groups were required to exercise, but whey protein still led to weight and fat loss. It is likely that anyone starting protein pacing will see similar benefits just from adding a whey protein supplement to their diet.

CHAPTER 4

THE BENEFITS OF PROTEIN PACING WITH EXERCISE

We've already seen how protein pacing can be beneficial for weight loss and losing body fat. A lot of other diets also make the same claims, so what makes this diet so special? The benefits of protein pacing go beyond just weight loss; it can improve your workout and a number of fitness measures as well, including improved upper body, lower body, and core strength, as well as improved balance and flexibility, increased power, and increased endurance.

There were two studies done that focused on protein pacing and exercise, called the PRISE II and PRISE III studies, both led by Dr. Paul Arciero of the original PRISE study. Let's look at both individually, as they deal with different groups of people. The PRISE II study looked at protein pacing in overweight men and women, and the PRISE III looked at women who were already physically active.

Whey Protein vs. Food Sources (the PRISE II Study)

Much like the first PRISE study, the PRISE II study included both protein pacing and an exercise program for the participants. In this study, which lasted 16 weeks, researchers also compared the effects of consuming whey protein with consuming protein-rich foods. Participants were all overweight or obese and led sedentary lifestyles. As a reminder, the important diet and exercise components of PRISE are protein pacing, resistance exercise, interval training, stretching/yoga/Pilates, and endurance exercise.

The study participants were divided into two groups. Those in the first group were required to eat five to six meals each day, with each meal consisting of 20 to 25 grams of protein. Whey protein supplements, also containing 20 to 25 grams of protein, would replace two of those meals every day, and on days that participants performed exercise, they would consume a third protein supplement in place of a meal, about one hour after exercising.

The second group was also required to eat five to six high-protein meals a day, each consisting of 20 to 25 grams of protein. These participants did not take protein supplements. They were encouraged to eat high-quality protein sources, including lean meats, fish, poultry, eggs, dairy products (such as milk or Greek yogurt), legumes, nuts, and seeds.

Both groups were required to participate in a varied exercise routine, which included the four different types of exercise typical to a PRISE study. Each exercise type was performed one day each week for less than an hour at a time, for a total of four days of exercise. For the interval training and endurance exercises, participants could select the activity of their choice.

For the participants in this study, protein intake was spaced out evenly throughout the day. One meal had to be eaten within one hour of waking, and the last meal of the day had to be eaten within two hours of bedtime. Participants were also required to have a meal or protein supplement (depending on the group) within one hour of exercising.

This study looked at body weight and total body composition, typical intake, and feelings of hunger. Blood was taken to check a lipid panel, as well as leptin, adiponectin, and insulin levels. The research team measured participants' resting energy expenditure, heart rate, and blood pressure. To check for any changes in fitness levels, participants also measured their upper and lower body strength, upper body endurance, core strength, balance, lower back flexibility, hamstring flexibility, and hand grip strength.

Participants in the study received online content that helped them maintain their program and diet. They were given diet and exercise information that they had learned previously, but having access to it reinforced previous teaching and helped them retain information. Having ready access to information can be particularly helpful for anyone trying to make diet and lifestyle changes, as it can help with retaining what you have learned, although you should make sure you are looking at a reputable source.

Although this was a small study of 21 participants, the results were very encouraging and consistent with the other protein pacing studies.

Study Results

Decreased body fat and weight. Both groups in the study lost weight, and both groups showed improvement in measurements of their waist circumference and a reduction in dangerous abdominal fat. There was not a significant difference in how much weight was lost between the supplement group or the high-protein food group. Over the time of the study, which was about four months, the average change in weight was about 4.8 kilograms (slightly over 10 pounds). Additionally, both groups saw a significant improvement in lean body mass.

Increased fitness. Both the whey protein supplement group and the high-protein food group had an improvement in all the fitness measures that were tracked. The most significant improvements were in upper and lower body strength, but both groups also improved in grip and core strength, upper body endurance, balance, and flexibility. Also, the resting energy expenditure (REE) went down for both groups. REE refers to how many calories we need during resting conditions, which is affected by a person's weight. It would make sense that REE would decrease, since total body weight had also gone down. REE tends to decrease when you lose weight, so you are burning fewer calories overall. Since you are burning less calories, this can make it more difficult to lose weight and keep it off.

Improved blood tests. Both groups tended to have a decrease in systolic heart rate. There was no change in heart rate or diastolic blood pressure. Blood tests showed that there were significant improvements in cholesterol levels, low-density lipoprotein (LDL) levels, triglycerides, blood sugar, insulin, leptin, and adiponectin. There were no changes in high-density lipoprotein (HDL) levels or estimated insulin resistance for either group.

Dietary changes. Protein intake significantly increased for both groups, while total carbohydrate intake decreased across the board. There were no changes in the total fat, fiber, or omega 3 fatty acid intake. Both groups reported feeling less hunger and had significant increases in satiety levels. As far as still feeling a desire to eat, which has a large psychological component, there was no real change.

Protein Pacing and Exercise in Women (PRISE III)

While the study above included people who led sedentary or inactive lifestyles, this study was done with women who were already physically active. This time, while all the women were engaged in the same varied exercise program, half of the participants would be eating their normal diets. The other half of the group would be protein pacing and consuming 2 grams of protein per kilogram body weight per day, which is about 0.9 grams of protein per pound.

Both groups in this study were eating the same number of calories and had their meals spaced out and timed so they were eating every three hours. The only difference between the two groups was how much protein they were consuming per day. Again, the results of this study confirmed the benefits of protein pacing, especially when combined with a highly varied exercise program.

Both groups saw improvements for all the fitness parameters being measured. Core strength and upper body muscle endurance were improved, more so in the group that was protein pacing. There was a big improvement in muscle power due to the exercise training, but it was greater in the group with the higher protein diet. Both groups also had an equal improvement in flexibility and balance.

Additionally, for both groups, there was a significant change in body composition during the study. Lean body mass percentage increased, and abdominal and hip fat decreased. Both systolic and diastolic blood pressures improved, but there was a greater improvement in the protein group. There was no difference in heart rate after the study.

While this study showed that a well-rounded exercise program could greatly improve someone's exercise performance, the biggest improvements were seen in the group that consumed a high-protein diet spaced evenly throughout the day. Not only was there an improvement in their fitness ability, but they had more noticeable changes in their body composition, as well.

Protein Pacing and Exercise in Men (Ives Study)

Like the women's study, research was also done on a group of male participants to examine the benefits of protein pacing and exercise in males, headed by Stephen Ives. Although this was not labeled a PRISE study, they also participated in many different types of exercises like those in the PRISE studies. The men in this study were divided into two groups: the protein pacing and exercise group, and the normal protein and exercise group. Those in the protein pacing group consumed 2 grams of protein per kilogram body weight spaced out throughout the day, while the normal protein group was only eating 1 gram of protein per kilogram each day. This would be equal to about 0.9 grams per pound and 0.45 grams per pound, respectively. The exercise program was the same for all the men involved, and the meal plans contained the same number of calories. Like in the PRISE studies, the men performed resistance exercise; interval training; stretching, yoga, or Pilates; and endurance exercise for one day each week, for a total of four days of exercise.

This study also had a specific regimen for meal timing and frequency. Prior to participating in resistance exercise or interval training, the men had a small snack, while they fasted for several hours prior to doing endurance exercise or stretching. Breakfast was eaten after the training session was complete. However, on days when the men were not exercising, they had to eat breakfast within an hour of waking. No matter what their breakfast time for each day in the study, the other meals were all spaced three hours apart.

Much like the PRISE III study, the protein pacing group had greater improvements in their physical fitness levels. Both groups had changes in body composition, including an increase in lean body mass and a loss of total body fat, abdominal fat, and hip fat. There was an improvement in core strength and upper body endurance in both groups, which was likely due to the exercise program. Both upper and lower body strength improved, but there was a greater improvement in upper body strength in the protein pacing group. There was also a noticeable improvement in both upper and lower body power, but the protein pacing group saw a bigger difference in lower body power. The men's flexibility levels improved over the course of the study, but more so in the protein pacing group. Both groups also improved at completing exercises when being timed, but the protein pacing group had a more significant improvement.

Systolic blood pressure improved in both groups, but there was no difference in diastolic blood pressure. Over the course of the study, the men's resting heart rate significantly reduced. Both groups in this study had an increase in their HDL cholesterol because of the exercise program, but changes were similar across groups.

Takeaways

The results of the PRISE II study are exciting, since they show that protein pacing can lead to improvements in overall fitness, no matter if you are taking a whey protein supplement or eating high-protein foods. These benefits can improve a person's ability to work out, which in turn can lead to further weight loss. Increased ability to exercise combined with weight loss will also lead to further improvements in overall health and well-being.

It can be daunting to start an intensive exercise program, especially if you have never done so before. However, the greatest benefits from protein pacing are shown when people also engage in a varied exercise program. Even though protein pacing has many benefits without exercising, you will have greater results in a shorter time frame if you begin a simple exercise program.

Both the PRISE III and Ives studies are important because they show how protein pacing can help improve physical fitness, on top of any other health or weight-loss goals. This is one of the benefits of protein pacing, and demonstrates just how multipurpose this way of eating can be.

Protein pacing is not something that should be limited to people who want to lose weight. Anyone who is looking to improve their overall fitness level and capabilities should try it, as well. It can also be looked at as a diet that can be adapted with your goals. It can be used for weight loss, and then when your goal weight is achieved, protein pacing can be continued to help you continue to make improvements with your exercise ability.

CHAPTER 5

PROTEIN PACING AND LONG-TERM WEIGHT LOSS

One of the most important things about a diet or lifestyle change is the ability to maintain weight loss. But it's not easy. People can lose a lot of weight fairly quickly, depending on how much weight they have to lose, but eventually, they get to a point where the weight loss will start to slow down, and then stop. This is known as a weight-loss plateau.

Why does this happen? When someone loses weight, they burn fewer calories than they did when they were at a heavier weight. If, now that they weigh less and are burning fewer calories, they are still eating the same number of calories as when they started to diet, then the weight loss will stop. When you hit a plateau, you need to either change the amount that you are eating or increase your exercise to continue to lose weight.

Weight-loss plateaus can cause a lot of frustration and lead to giving up. Once they hit a plateau, many people may start to regain the weight that they lost, and it may be a while before they attempt to lose weight again. Or, some people may look to other, unsafe methods to try and speed up the weight-loss process.

A study was done to address how well protein pacing would affect people's ability to maintain weight loss. The thought behind the study is that protein pacing would help with weight maintenance because of the thermic effect of food: There would be an increased energy expenditure, which would hopefully prevent a decrease in metabolism.

In this next study, also led by Paul Arciero, protein pacing was studied over the course of more than a year to see if it would result in successful weight maintenance. The study was separated into two time frames: a three-month weight-loss phase, followed by a one-year weight-management phase.

For the first three months of the study, all the people participating followed a protein pacing and calorie-restricted diet. Everyone was also assigned to see a registered dietitian on a weekly basis. During this phase, for six days each week, breakfast and lunch were limited to a meal replacement shake that had 240 calories and 24 grams of protein. Men were allowed a 150-calorie afternoon snack and a 600-calorie dinner, while women did not have an afternoon snack and were allotted 450 calories for dinner. This difference was because men generally have higher calorie needs than women. Everyone was allowed an evening snack bar that contained 250 calories and 18 grams of protein. Over the course of a day, men consumed about 1,500 calories and women ate about 1,200 calories.

On the seventh day, all the people in the study were then required to participate in intermittent fasting, an eating pattern where you cycle through periods of eating and periods of fasting. Women were limited to 350 calories on this day, while men could eat 450 calories.

During the remaining nine months of the study, half of the subjects followed a modified protein pacing diet while the other half followed a heart healthy diet. Interestingly, people were allowed to select whether they wanted to follow a protein pacing or heart healthy diet for this second part of the study. This probably helped with compliance, because everyone was following the diet of their choice. Additionally, participants followed up with their dietitian monthly to help maintain their eating choices. Depending on the person, they could have additional visits if needed.

Participants who chose protein pacing would eat four to five meals per day, with two of those meals consumed as protein shakes or bars. The other two or three meals were made up of real food of any type. There was still intermittent fasting, but now it occurred only once or twice a month instead of every week. Those who chose to participate in the heart healthy group followed a diet that contained less than 35 percent of calories from fat, 50 to 60 percent of calories from carbohydrates, less than 200 mg/dL of cholesterol, and at least 20 grams of fiber per day. These participants also followed a pattern of intermittent fasting.

To make the research study more realistic and sustainable, participants weren't restricted on their food intake or physical activity during this phase. Otherwise, if they were given very strict meal plans or had their meals provided, the results would not necessarily be true to life. This study was meant to show whether protein pacing could be used for successful weight maintenance while people were living their normal lives.

Weight-Loss Phase Results

The weight loss and change in body composition after the weight-loss phase is impressive and reinforces the results from prior studies on the benefits of protein pacing.

Reduced dietary intake. On the initial diet, the total daily intake for men and women was reduced by 50 percent. Participants were eating 12 to 15 percent less fat than they had previously, and their carbohydrate intake was close to half of what it was previously. Protein intake obviously significantly increased. The initial diet also led to an increase in dietary fiber and a decreased intake of sugar and sodium. Even though there was a significant difference in caloric intake, there was no change in feelings of hunger and satiety.

Changes in body weight and body composition. During the weight-loss phase, both men and women lost just over 10 percent of their total body weight. On average, they also lost 19 percent total body fat and 25 percent of their abdominal fat. There was also a decrease in total lean body mass (on average, about 4 pounds), likely due to the calorie restriction. However, even though there was a decrease in lean body mass, the total proportion of lean body mass actually increased, if we look at body composition as a whole. Additionally, during the weight-loss phase, participants showed a relative improvement in resting metabolic rate (RMR), measured by looking at the number of calories burned per kilogram of body weight. This is likely because the protein pacing led to increased proportion of lean body mass, one of the main things that can affect our RMR.

Reduced blood sugar levels. Fasting blood sugar dropped for both men and women. A decrease in insulin was noted as well.

Leptin levels decreased by over 50 percent in men and nearly 75 percent in women, but adiponectin levels did not change during this phase of the diet.

Weight-Maintenance Phase Results

Increased hunger. Both groups had increased hunger levels and a greater desire to eat by the end of the study, though there were no differences between the intake of the two groups except for the fact that the heart healthy group was consuming more sodium. There was no change in blood sugar and insulin levels for either group by the end of the study. Leptin and adiponectin levels had only been checked midway through the study and not at the end, but levels had increased in both groups.

Weight gain. Both groups in this study ended up gaining some weight back and seeing an increase in waist circumference. Both traits were seen less in the protein pacing group than in the heart healthy group.

The heart healthy group had a bigger change in their total percentage of body fat. This group ended up gaining body fat, while the protein pacing group had a slight loss. There was also an increase in percentage of abdominal fat and total fat, and a loss of lean body mass in the heart healthy group. The protein pacing group had a similar amount of abdominal fat compared with the heart healthy group. However, they began this portion of the study with a slight gain in lean body mass, and only a slight gain in fat mass, meaning their gain was still less than that of the heart healthy group.

Takeaways

Following a lower calorie diet has been proven to result in weight loss. For obvious reasons, if we eat fewer calories than we are burning, our bodies will need to break down fat and muscle to produce the energy that we need. However, in many cases, very few people can keep up with the diet in the long term and end up gaining a lot of weight back. Hormones are another possible cause of weight regain. As necessary as hormones are, they don't always act in a way that we would like. Some hormones that have roles in affecting our body weight may end up leading us to gain weight back.

Not only did this study reinforce the fact that protein pacing is an effective way to lose weight and change your overall body composition, but it showed that it was something that could be maintained over a long period of time. The protein pacing group in this study had body weight gain of less than 1 percent after the initial weight-loss phase, while the heart healthy group had more than a 6 percent weight gain.

Another positive to note in this study is that even though there was a loss in lean body mass after the weight-loss phase, the percentage of lean body mass actually increased for those who participated in the protein pacing plan. Even with the slight loss, it is still better to have a higher percentage of lean body mass compared to having a higher percentage from fat. The protein pacing group also maintained the loss of total body fat and abdominal body fat. As discussed before, abdominal fat can have a lot of negative effects on our health, so being able to lose it and keep it off is extremely important.

Protein Pacing and Long-Term Weight Loss

Research also shows how the overall diet quality is important. Even though both groups in this study saw a lot of positive benefits from the initial weight loss, only the protein pacing group maintained those benefits. It was not that the heart healthy group was eating a lot more calories; actually, there were not that many differences except for the fact that they had a higher salt intake. But they ended up gaining back a lot more weight and body fat. We can see from other studies that it is very difficult to prevent gaining weight back when there is not enough protein included in the diet.

This study suggests that protein pacing is a beneficial program for long-term weight loss because of its effects on appetite and satiety. Protein foods can help you feel fuller longer than if you had a low-protein meal with the same number of calories. And when you include protein in your diet regularly, it helps delay feelings of hunger. Feelings of satiety and hunger can greatly affect someone's weight-loss progress and their ability to stick to a program. Hunger is an unpleasant sensation that can lead to feelings of deprivation, which can lead to overeating or binge eating.

Although we obviously eat for a lot of reasons besides actually being hungry, someone's desire to eat can be affected by several psychological factors as well, such as mood, the environment, and who you spend time with. It is likely that over the duration of this year-long study, there would have been many opportunities for a participant to eat other than hunger. This is normal in day-to-day life, and it is not realistic to think that we can live our lives like a science experiment. The fact is that the people in the protein pacing group were able to maintain their weight loss when going about their normal lives despite all the other things that could have affected what they were eating. This reinforces the idea that protein pacing is the type of diet plan that can work in the real world and will actually produce sustainable weight loss, unlike many other fad diets.

PART 2
THE DIET

CHAPTER 6

MY EXPERIENCE WITH PROTEIN PACING

I did not feel like I could recommend protein pacing unless I had tried it myself. This is like something I did back when I was in college, when I would have to follow specialized diet plans for classes so that I could see what it was like for people with different medical conditions and dietary restrictions. It was not always easy, and it made me realize why people are not always compliant with following their diet.

After completing my research for this book, I was confident that I would not have any issues following a protein pacing plan myself. I decided to conduct my own mini–protein pacing research study over a five-week period. I was interested in seeing what changes would happen to my body, and if I would notice any of the stated benefits of taking whey protein or following a protein pacing meal pattern.

Preparing for Protein Pacing

While I am at a healthy weight for my height and have a normal BMI, I did anticipate seeing some weight loss given the study results discussed in the previous chapters. However, I also wanted to increase my muscle mass and improve my strength. A lot of the activities that I enjoy doing, such as indoor rock climbing and kayaking, require a lot of upper body strength, and women tend to have less upper body strength than men do. On days that I am really trying to push myself, I find that I get tired very easily.

To collect as much starting information on myself as I could, I checked my weight, body fat, and muscle mass on body fat scales that would calculate this information. Now, these types of scales are known to be inaccurate, and the results can be affected by a number of things. Even if your feet are wet, it could produce a different result. For the sake of this study, I checked my weight, body fat, and muscle mass percentage on three different scales. Many home scales now come with these options.

Besides the scale measurements, I also used a tape measure to take measurements of my waist circumference, legs, and upper arms to see if those numbers would be affected over time. This experiment has limitations, because there is no way to tell exactly what would cause changes in waist, leg, or arm size; it only tracks whether changes occur, and to what extent. However, taking these measurements is still a good way to check if you are making progress, especially if your body weight remains the same. I was careful to document where exactly I was taking my measurements to make sure I measured the same place before and after my experiment.

Even though the benefits of protein pacing can be seen without exercise, I kept to my regular exercise regimen for the duration of my experiment because I did not want to change my baseline activity level. Much of my exercise comes from walking, and as I mentioned before, I do enjoy some other athletic activities. If I had changed my workout routine at all, that could have affected my results. I wanted to make sure that the results I saw were simply from the addition of whey protein. As far as my regular diet, I tend to follow a fairly healthful diet, since I am a dietitian and I believe in practicing what I preach.

To see if I felt any changes in hunger or satiety, or to see if protein pacing would affect how much I was eating of any particular food groups, I started a food diary prior to starting the experiment. I filled out the food diary for seven days before starting protein pacing, and then for three days each week (two weekdays and one weekend day). For the entire last week of my experiment, I kept a food diary as well. I kept everything written down in a small notebook that I carried around with me, just so I would remember to record everything.

The Experiment

I decided that I would split this experiment up into two separate parts. In the first part, I would take the whey protein supplement two or three times a day, depending on whether I was getting any real physical activity in, such as yoga, running, or indoor rock climbing. This was modeled after the PRISE I and PRISE II studies, and I wanted to make sure that I was taking the protein supplement after exercise to provide the amino acids I needed for muscle building and recovery.

To start my day, I drank the whey protein supplement within one hour of getting up in the morning. The whey supplement that I used had 120 calories and 24 grams of protein per serving, which was pretty close to what the participants in the studies used. It also had a small amount of fat (2 grams) and carbohydrates (3 grams). The only ingredient in the product was whey protein isolate. If I was participating in some sort of physical activity, I would have another whey supplement within an hour of completing the exercise. I tried to drink it as soon as I could after I was done working out, but if I was driving home and did not have it with me, it sometimes took a little longer. My last dose of the whey supplement was at night, usually about an hour before I went to bed.

I mixed the supplement with about 10 ounces of water, as I found this was an amount that mixed well without producing a strong taste. One thing that I noticed right away is that even though I had bought unflavored whey protein powder, it still had a very mild taste. I did not find the taste to be bad; I just wasn't expecting to taste it at all. It almost tastes like very watered-down skim milk, which makes sense, since it is derived from cow's milk.

I also found that I did not take the supplement unless it was convenient, time-wise. Initially when I started protein pacing, I planned on taking a mid-afternoon dose of the whey supplement, even if I was not exercising. I tried bringing the powder to work, but because I run around the majority of the day, I never got to drink it. Also, one day I had whey protein powder in a plastic baggie in my lab coat pocket, and I ended up ripping it open, which caused a giant mess. Usually by the time I left work and got home, it was close to dinner time, and I did not want to take the protein supplement right before dinner, as it would affect my appetite too much. After that, I decided to take the whey supplement twice a day unless I was exercising, in which case I would take it three times.

During the second part of my experience, I changed the way I eat so that I was eating five or six meals a day, and I tried not to use protein supplements unless I really did not have access to real food. Each meal and snack needed to include 20 to 25 grams of protein. This was the more challenging part of protein pacing, as it required me to prepare my meals and snacks in advance. I found this more difficult when I was going out to eat or planned to be out of the house for most of the day. If I was not sure that I would be able to stop somewhere to pick up a snack or find an appropriate meal, I brought food with me in an insulated lunch box. This required a lot more planning, but it was doable if I prepared foods in bulk on slower days. On some days when I was really busy, I just drank a whey protein supplement since it was much easier than cooking or carrying food around.

The Experience

Based on the research I'd read, it appeared that protein pacing would be able to yield very impressive results from a very simple intervention. I am glad that I tried out both methods, but I much preferred taking the whey protein supplement because it was easier than having to prepare so many appropriate meals and snacks. I would recommend adding whey protein supplements to someone interested in trying protein pacing, just because of the amount of work involved. If they have time, they could move onto the meal preparation style of protein pacing.

The first part of my protein pacing plan was extremely simple: I was just adding a whey protein supplement twice daily (three times on days with exercise). I found that adding the protein supplement worked well with my lifestyle, as it required very little preparation on my part and I did not feel like I needed to overhaul my diet. This simpler version of the diet may be more realistic for most people. If I told everyone they needed to eat 20 to 25 grams of protein per meal and space those meals out evenly through the day, a lot less people would be willing to try it or able to comply.

The most important question is, was I able to be compliant? For much of the time, yes. There were a few evenings where I had events to go to and I ended up getting home late, so I skipped the evening protein supplement on a few days or wasn't sure if the meal I was eating actually had 25 grams of protein. Another time, I had a mid-morning wedding and I wanted to enjoy the wedding food, so I was not compliant on that day, either. But overall, I consumed the protein supplement and followed the meal plans for more than 90 percent of the time. Obviously, no one can be perfect all the time, and things do happen that can throw off our plans, but for the most part, I was easily able to make protein pacing work with my lifestyle.

Results

Satiety. Protein pacing did affect my appetite, especially in the morning and later in the evenings when I would typically have a snack. Prior to starting protein pacing, I would normally be starving by the time I got to work and want to eat breakfast right away, but once I started drinking the supplement, I noticed almost immediately that I was not hungry when I got to work. I started eating my breakfast in the morning later than I normally had, usually around 10:00 instead of around 7:00 or 8:00. I was also getting full before I finished my meal, which I would easily eat all of before I started protein pacing. Since I was eating breakfast later in the morning, I found that I did not need to have a mid-morning snack as I typically would. When I took the afternoon protein supplement, I wasn't as hungry at dinner and often could not finish all of my meal.

The last whey protein supplement I would take was within two hours of bedtime, after dinner. After drinking the protein supplement, I was not hungry at night for any other snacks. Before protein pacing, I would eat refined carbohydrates and less healthy snacks later in the evening, but after I started protein pacing, I pretty much stopped having any other sort of food in the evening, as I just wasn't hungry for it. There were times that I was not even hungry for the protein supplement or bar, but I would take it anyway to be more compliant with the diet.

Daily intake. While I have always had a healthful diet, I noticed that protein pacing really changed my daily intake. There wasn't too much of a significant difference in my total calorie intake over the course of the experiment: Drinking the whey protein supplement or having supplements and a protein bar added at least another 240 calories to my day (or 360 calories, if I had a third supplement after exercising), but I was eating less at meals. My food diary near the end of the experiment showed that I had been consuming an average of 50 calories less per day than before I started protein pacing because I was eating less food from meals and snacks, despite the extra calories from supplements.

The biggest difference was in the macronutrients that I was eating. My intake of protein was obviously much higher, and I was taking in fewer carbohydrates overall. I was specifically eating fewer refined carbohydrates and sugars. Since I mainly ate these foods at snack times, my intake of refined carbohydrates was cut out almost completely. These are the foods that really aren't necessary in the diet at all anyway, and I try to limit them since they tend to provide calories and sugar without a lot of other nutrients. While I was protein pacing, I found that it was pretty easy to give up these foods.

I also drank a lot more water during this time. Not only was I getting some extra fluid with the protein supplement, but I made a point to try and drink more water, as higher protein intake can lead to dehydration if you are not drinking enough. This can be dangerous during the summertime or when you are exercising. I typically drink around 70 to 80 ounces per day, but I increased my water intake to at least 100 ounces per day while protein pacing.

Body composition. At the end of the five-week period, I checked my weight, body fat, and muscle mass percentage on the same three scales that I had initially used to try for the most accuracy. The numbers did vary slightly between scales, so I averaged the numbers from the beginning of the experiment and compared them to the numbers from the end of the experiment.

Before I weighed myself, I noticed that my pants fit slightly looser. The numbers confirmed that I had lost some weight: I lost a total of 3½ pounds, which I immediately thought would be all muscle loss since I had not increased my exercise routine at all. Surprisingly, it was not. My muscle mass percentage was fairly stable (it was within 0.5 percent from the start), but I had lost 2 percent body fat.

Aside from the scale numbers, I also took measurements of my waist circumference, legs, and upper arms. Interestingly, my upper arms were about ¼ inch larger at the end of my study, although this is not that significant and may have been due to where my arms were measured; I had to ask for assistance to take arm measurements. Even if this measurement was slightly off, it is likely that I did not lose much, if any, muscle in my arms. Since protein pacing requires higher protein intake, there should not be as much muscle loss as with typical dieting, even if you are not exercising. My waist circumference and legs had more noticeable results. I had lost an inch off my waist and hips, and slightly over an inch from my thighs. I am much more confident in these measurements than those of my arms, as I was able to do those measurements myself and know that I measured in the same spot.

Takeaways

Overall, I felt that my experiment was successful, and I can honestly say it was fairly easy to do. I did not feel put out by having to drink the protein supplement, and it worked well with my lifestyle. I really liked the fact that you can do a basic version of protein pacing with your normal diet that does not require a lot of meal prepping. It is a program that can be flexible depending on what is going on in your life.

For anyone looking to make additional lifestyle changes, I have included several healthful, high-protein recipes, many of which can be prepared ahead of time and then reheated, in Chapter 10.

CHAPTER 7

INCORPORATING EXERCISE

Even though protein pacing will help you lose weight on its own, any exercise program that you start will only help you lose more weight. In fact, as little as 20 minutes of moderate-level physical activity done most days of the week can increase your metabolism.

Exercising does not mean that you need to go to a gym and hire a personal trainer. Having a personal trainer can be a great option for some people, but it can also get really expensive. Depending on where you live or how long your commute is, going to a gym during the workday may not be possible. And while group exercise classes can be fun, they can also be intimidating if you haven't worked out before or if everyone else in the class has a higher fitness level than you. The point of starting an exercise program is not to compare yourself to others or to feel like you can't keep up. While I would definitely recommend exercising, you should make it as easy as possible to incorporate fitness into your life.

Do not feel that you necessarily need to start working out for an hour at a time. Making small changes to your day-to-day routine is the best way to lose weight and keep it off. For instance, take five minutes at the end of your lunch break to do some sit-to-stand transfers. You will get your heart rate up and it won't take a lot of time out of your day. Keep in mind that you can do whichever exercises appeal to you at whatever level you find comfortable. For example, if you model an exercise program after the PRISE studies, you may choose to try a yoga class one day, and then take a walk in a park on another day. The most important thing is that you are trying to incorporate different forms of exercise, even if you are not able to complete an entire hour.

Another benefit to having a varied exercise program is that it helps keep your interest and prevents you from getting burned out. How many people do you know that have signed up for a gym that only offers one type of class, just to quit a few weeks later? If you are feeling bored when you are exercising, you will be less likely to make an effort, which defeats the purpose of exercising in the first place. Including different types of exercise also works different muscles and keeps your body from getting used to a routine, which will help you keep seeing results. However, for anyone who has had a heart attack or a stroke, or has any other preexisting medical conditions, please discuss starting an exercise program with your primary care physician or cardiologist.

Resistance Training

Resistance training does not need to be done at a gym, and you don't even have to purchase any equipment. If you have never done any type of resistance training before, it is completely possible to get in a work out with items that you have around the house. If you have access to a backyard or a local park and are comfortable outdoors, you can even take the workout outside to make it more enjoyable. Resistance training is any type of training where you are using force against another object. Weight lifting would probably be the first thing that comes to mind, but you can also do exercises using your own body weight.

Weight-lifting moves can be done using common household items. You can start with a very light object and work your way up to something heavier (such as starting with a 16-ounce bottle of water, and then increasing to 24 ounces, and then 32 ounces, etc.). Canned goods and bottled beverages can be great for doing bicep curls, working on your triceps, and doing different shoulder exercises.

Using your own body weight is also a good way to do a resistance exercise. These types of exercises include push-ups, bear crawls, crunches, and sit-ups. For additional suggestions, a good reference is the American College for Sports Medicine website at ACSM.org, which provides educational information, links to blogs, and other educational materials.

Interval Training

Interval training refers to alternating very short periods of high-intensity activity with rest periods or exercises at a much lower intensity. Interval training has been found to burn more calories than if you were doing an exercise at the same intensity over a long period of time; it can also reduce waist circumference.

It also provides good exercise for the heart muscle, which can improve your aerobic capacity. Interval training can produce the same improvements in cardiovascular fitness as endurance training, but in a shorter amount of time. In general, interval training may be more effective at reducing body fat than endurance exercises.

One example of an interval training exercise would be a sit-to-stand transfer. Start in a sitting position on a sturdy chair or bench. For 30 seconds, stand up and sit down as many times as you can. Make sure to go at your own pace so that you feel comfortable. If you are not used to exercising and start to feel dizzy, slow down or take a break. When you have reached 30 seconds, rest for one minute. Repeat this routine, 30 seconds of activity followed by one minute of rest, for as long as you feel comfortable. Or before you start, decide on a goal of how many rounds you want to complete. This is a great way to build up your activity tolerance.

Jumping jacks, jumping rope, and marching in place are also good ways to do an interval training workout in the comfort and privacy of your own home. The most important thing is to go at your own pace. Either decide on a goal (such as getting through four rounds), or you can try to see how many you can do before you get tired.

Stretching, Yoga, and Pilates

Stretching, yoga, and Pilates are so important because these types of exercise help keep muscles long and flexible. Flexibility helps maintain range of motion within the joints, decreasing risk of joint strain or damage. These exercises are also good for improving balance, which can prevent injuries.

There are many great stretching, yoga, or Pilates programs that you can find online for free. Many videos are readily accessible via YouTube, and yogajournal.org is a great resource for different poses. If you are new to yoga and wanted to try it, I would suggest taking a few beginner classes at a studio to learn the proper positions and alignment. Many places are willing to offer coupons or specials to new members. Otherwise, you can find programs online, and frequently can read reviews from other people to determine if it is right for you. For any new stretching, yoga, or Pilates program, be careful to choose one that states that it is good for beginners. More advanced programs can be complicated, and you do not want to strain yourself if you are not at that fitness level yet. Examples of stretching, yoga, and Pilates positions include the runner's lunge, hamstring stretch, and quadriceps stretch.

Endurance Training

Endurance aerobic exercises are great for keeping your heart and lungs healthy, as well as improving your overall fitness level. The term aerobic simply means that the exercise requires oxygen. Regular aerobic activity will help strengthen the heart muscle and can help it pump more efficiently. Aerobic exercise can also strengthen the lungs and improve circulation. The benefits of aerobic exercise extend beyond the physical, as it can actually help improve mental health. You can choose whatever type of aerobic exercise you enjoy, as that will make you more likely to stick with it. To keep things more interesting, you can switch between activity types every few weeks, or even within the same training session if you prefer.

Aerobic activities are diverse and versatile. For example, any of the exercises you would do as an interval activity can also be used for an endurance exercise. You could also go on a walk, bike, or swim. Walking puts a lot less stress on the joints, biking activates many muscle groups, and swimming builds endurance and can help increase muscle strength, while taking more stress off the joints.

No matter what activity you decide to do, even slightly increasing your physical activity level can provide a number of health and wellness benefits. In the studies that I have reviewed, the participants got the most benefit from doing a highly varied exercise program. They would participate in one session of resistance training, interval workouts, stretching, yoga, or Pilates exercises, and endurance activities each week, which totals out to exercising on four days each week.

CHAPTER 8

START PROTEIN PACING

One of the best things about protein pacing is the variety of options for following the plan. The studies discussed in the previous chapters each included different versions of a protein pacing meal pattern, from some that were very simple to ones that got a little more complicated. In this section, I'll discuss the meal patterns that were used in the studies so that you can decide which one would be best for you.

The nice thing about protein pacing is that it can be flexible. If you decide to try eating multiple meals per day about three hours apart and it doesn't work for you, you shouldn't give up. You can always try switching to drinking a whey protein supplement twice a day, and keeping your normal diet, as that has also shown to have weight-loss benefits. If you don't want to start an exercise program at this time, you don't have to. Protein pacing is not like other diets where you need to only eat certain foods for two weeks, and then add in other foods. It doesn't force you to eliminate your favorite foods. In order to be successful with this type of meal plan, you need to figure out what is most realistic for you and what works with your lifestyle.

Option 1: Additional Protein Supplement

In the PRISE study, the first study discussed in this book, the participants who were protein pacing consumed an additional protein supplement every day in addition to eating their normal diets. This is a great place to start if you are ready to start protein pacing but aren't ready to make a lot of dietary changes. This study also showed that protein pacing was effective for weight loss and body composition changes, even without an exercise program. If you do choose to start an exercise program, you will see greater results, but it is not necessary.

If you are someone who has less time during the day, then using a whey protein supplement would be the best way to start protein pacing. You should pick a whey protein supplement that contains about 120 calories and 20 to 25 grams of protein per serving. When you are protein pacing, you will be drinking the whey protein supplement three times daily at specific times during the day. Even if you do not have time to exercise, you should see weight loss and a loss of total body fat (including abdominal fat) just by adding the whey protein supplement to your normal diet.

Dose 1: 1 serving of whey protein should be taken within one hour of waking up in the morning.

Dose 2: 1 serving of whey protein should be taken in the middle of the afternoon, or immediately after an exercise session.

Dose 3: 1 serving of whey protein should be taken within two hours of going to sleep.

This option is fairly easy and does not require significant work or changes. Of course, you will only see additional benefits from other diet and lifestyle changes, but this is a good starting place. You will see results just from adding the whey protein supplement to your normal diet.

Option 2: Protein Pacing and Meal Timing

While protein pacing with meal timing was done in conjunction with exercise for the Ives study on page 42, you should still see results even if you are not participating in an exercise program. Having regular meals with a good source of protein at each meal will help keep your metabolism up, and you should not feel hungry since protein helps increase satiety.

If you choose this option and do not want to take the supplement at the specified meal times, it is okay to switch it with another meal. The only requirements are the timing of the meals and the amount of protein that they must contain. No calorie counting is required, and there are no other food restrictions.

This would be a great option for someone who does not want to rely on protein supplements, or who enjoys cooking and preparing meals. I would suggest creating a menu for at least a week at a time, and trying to prepare what you can in advance to make it easier to stick with. And even if you are not able to prepare five or six meals per day, the whey supplement is an easy option as a backup.

I have included sample meal times to show you how the meals might be spaced out, and how you might incorporate the protein supplement. That does not mean that you need to have meals at these particular times. No matter if you get up earlier or later, you should still have your first meal of the day within one hour of waking up.

SAMPLE PROTEIN PACING & MEAL-TIMING SCHEDULE	
MEAL TIME	MEAL REQUIREMENTS
6:00 a.m. *within 1 hour of rising*	Whey protein supplement or meal that contains 20–25 grams protein
9:00 a.m., mid-morning meal *3 hours after first meal*	Meal must contain 20–25 grams high biological value protein
12:00 p.m., lunch meal *3 hours after mid-morning meal*	Meal must contain 20–25 grams high biological value protein
3:00 p.m., mid-afternoon meal *3 hours after lunch*	Whey protein supplement or meal that contains 20–25 grams protein
6:00 p.m., dinner meal, *3 hours after mid-afternoon meal*	Meal must contain 20–25 grams high biological value protein
9:30 p.m., pre-bedtime meal *should be taken about 3 hours after dinner meal but must be consumed within 2 hours of bedtime*	Meal must contain 20–25 grams high biological value protein

Option 3: Meal Planning, Protein Pacing, and Meal Timing with Exercise

The study of protein pacing in exercising men (page 42) set forth a specific diet schedule depending on the type of activity being undertaken that day. Although this study was specifically done on men, it is a program that would be beneficial for women, as well. This is the type of protein pacing meal pattern that you should follow if you were also participating in a highly varied exercise program that included resistance exercise, interval training, endurance activity, and stretching, Pilates, or yoga. Remember that in the studies, each of the types of exercise were done one day each week, for a total of four exercise days.

Since this meal plan was used in a study that showed the effects of protein pacing on fitness, you would want to follow the example of the non-exercise days if you are not starting an exercise program. While the chart indicates that you should eat six meals per day, this can be adjusted to be five or six meals depending on your preference and appetite.

MEAL PLANNING, PROTEIN PACING, & EXERCISE		
ACTIVITY	BREAKFAST MEAL REQUIREMENTS	OTHER MEAL REQUIREMENTS
Non-exercise days	Breakfast must be consumed within 1 hour of waking up	All of the five remaining meals must be consumed every three hours after the breakfast meal
Resistance training	No normal breakfast meal, small snack consumed prior to exercise	Meal consumed after exercise, all remaining meals must be consumed every three hours after post-exercise meal
Interval training	No normal breakfast meal, small snack consumed prior to exercise	Meal consumed after exercise, all remaining meals must be consumed every three hours after post-exercise meal
Stretching, yoga, or Pilates	No breakfast meal, must fast for several hours prior to activity	Meal consumed after exercise, all remaining meals must be consumed every three hours after post-exercise meal

If you choose to follow this pattern of protein pacing, you should be eating 2 grams of protein per kilogram per day. In order to figure out how many grams of protein you need, you will first need to determine your weight in kilograms (1 kilogram is equal to 2.2 pounds).

When you figure out how much protein you should have each day, it should be spaced out evenly throughout the day at all meals, unless there is a specific meal requirement listed prior to exercise.

For example, if someone weighs 150 pounds, that is equal to about 68 kilograms. For them to follow this type of meal pattern, they would need to eat 136 grams of protein each day (68 kilograms x 2 grams per kilogram of protein = 136 grams of protein). Spacing this out evenly throughout the day, they would need to eat 22 to 27 grams of protein at each meal time.

Option 4: Protein Pacing with Calorie Restriction for Weight Loss

This version of protein pacing is very different from the ones prior, as it also includes intermittent fasting, like in the study discussed on page 48. Intermittent fasting has been gaining more interest due to the belief that it can help you live longer and reduce the risks of diseases that are common in the elderly (although more research is needed in this subject area). There is also some thought that it can help burn body fat faster, but again, this area needs more research. Intermittent fasting is not appropriate for someone who has diabetes, due to the risk of low blood sugar, especially if you are taking oral medications or are on insulin. If you are a diabetic and want to follow a protein pacing, calorie-restricted diet, you may be able to do so if you do not partake in intermittent fasting. I would advise to talk about this with your physician.

If you choose to try a protein pacing, calorie-restricted diet, this type of plan will require more preparation since you need to restrict your total intake, unlike with some of the other studies, which only had the requirement that you needed to eat a certain amount of protein. You cannot just eat whatever you want for dinner; you need to portion out your ingredients to stick to the allowed calorie level. It also includes meal replacement shakes. You can purchase premade shakes that have a similar calorie and protein content to the ones used in the study, or you can make your own at home using the whey protein powder.

Premade shakes should not be used for the other protein pacing options, as they can provide excess calories. They are acceptable in this type of plan as they are used as a meal replacement. Men and women choosing this type of meal pattern will have different diets due to the different calorie levels that have been assigned.

In the study reviewed on page 48, the protein pacing with calorie restriction phase of the diet went on for three months prior to switching to the weight-maintenance phase of the diet. This would be an appropriate time frame to follow, as well. However, you can always return to this phase of the diet if you decide that you want to lose more weight later.

THE PROTEIN PACING DIET

On one day each week, you would partake in intermittent fasting (though see note above about consulting with a physician). On the intermittent fasting day, you must limit your intake to no more than 350 calories for women and 450 calories for men. If you prefer to drink a protein supplement on this day you can, or you can consume snacks made from real foods.

PROTEIN PACING WITH CALORIE RESTRICTION FOR WOMEN*	
MEAL TIME	MEAL REQUIREMENTS
Breakfast	Meal replacement shake *containing 240 calories and 24 grams protein*
Lunch	Meal replacement shake *containing 240 calories and 24 grams protein*
Mid-afternoon snack	No afternoon snack allowed
Dinner	Meal prepared from whole food ingredients *450 calories, no specified protein requirement*
Evening snack	Protein snack bar *containing 250 calories and 18 grams protein*

* Limited to 1,200 calories per day, 6 days each week

PROTEIN PACING WITH CALORIE RESTRICTION FOR MEN*	
MEAL TIME	MEAL REQUIREMENTS
Breakfast	Meal replacement shake *containing 240 calories and 24 grams protein*
Lunch	Meal replacement shake *containing 240 calories and 24 grams protein*
Mid-afternoon snack	whole foods or snack bar allowed *150 calories, no specified protein requirement*
Dinner	Meal prepared from whole food ingredients *600 calories, no specified protein requirement*
Evening snack	Protein snack bar *containing 250 calories and 18 grams protein*

* Limited to 1,500 calories per day, 6 days each week

Option 5: Protein Pacing for Long-Term Weight Maintenance

This version of protein pacing should be used after you have already lost the amount of weight that you desire and are ready to start a maintenance plan. This plan will allow you to sustain your results without worrying about gaining back a significant amount of weight.

The table below shows a basic meal pattern for this phase of the diet. Based on the study on page 48, the requirements of this phase were that two high-protein meal replacements had to be eaten or drunk each day. This was either two protein shakes, or one protein shake and a meal replacement bar. You were not required to eat these products at any specific meals, so the meal slots that I put them in can be moved around, depending on what works best with your lifestyle. The meals were also not required to be eaten at any specific time, so there is more flexibility in this diet. However, even though there is not a set schedule for the meals, I would still suggest trying to space them out evenly throughout the day.

The protein shake and protein bar do vary in the number of calories that they contain. Numbers in the charts below reflect the calorie and protein counts from the products that were available to the study participants. While choosing a protein shake or bar, you should aim for a product containing around 250 calories and 18 to 24 grams of protein.

PROTEIN PACING FOR LONG-TERM WEIGHT MAINTENANCE	
MEAL NUMBER	MEAL REQUIREMENTS
Meal 1 *no set time for consumption*	Protein shake containing about 240 calories and 24 grams of protein
Meal 2 *no set time for consumption*	Meal to be made up of real food, no restrictions on calories or type of food consumed
Meal 3 *no set time for consumption*	Meal to be made up of real food, no restrictions on calories or type of food consumed
Meal 4 *no set time for consumption*	Must either drink a protein shake containing about 240 calories and 24 grams of protein, or eat a protein bar containing around 250 calories and 18 grams of protein
Meal 5 *no set time for consumption*	Meal to be made up of real food, no restrictions on calories or type of food consumed

Even though this was the weight-maintenance phase of the study, intermittent fasting is still required. Instead of fasting every week, you should be intermittently fasting for only one or two days each month. On fasting days, you should stick to the calorie restrictions from the weight-loss phase. Men should eat no more than 450 calories, and women are limited to 350 calories on intermittent fasting days.

The purpose of providing you with the different meal patterns that were followed in the studies is to give you options on how to follow a protein pacing diet. The research that has been done so far on this topic shows the benefits of protein pacing and how it has been used in many ways. There is a way to protein pace that will maximize exercise benefits, and another that will lead to weight loss followed by weight maintenance. Most importantly, there is a very simple version of a protein pacing diet that can be followed if you have been struggling with losing weight and aren't ready to make significant dietary changes. Having this type of flexibility in the program is what makes protein pacing successful. When there are options that are realistic for your everyday life, you are more likely to stick with the program, which is really how we can define success.

Tips for Protein Pacing

It can be frustrating to start a new diet or exercise program and not lose weight. If you are losing body fat and gaining muscle mass, you may not necessarily see a change in the number on the scale. That is why other measurements, such as body fat and percentage of muscle mass, are so important to help judge your progress. I would recommend taking these three measurements before you begin protein pacing, even if the scales you use are not completely accurate. This can be helpful to give you an idea of your progress. You may also notice differences in how your clothes fit and how you feel. I do have one suggestion for anyone taking measurements prior to starting any sort of weight-loss plan. It can be very difficult to make sure that you are measuring in the same place, but if you have any birthmarks or freckles, these can be used as "markers" so you know you are in the same location.

I also recommend tracking your food intake for at least a few days prior to starting protein pacing, and then keeping up with it for the first few weeks. This would be especially helpful if you are not familiar with how many calories and how much protein are in the foods you normally eat. If you prefer not to use a notebook, there are a lot of apps where you can record your food intake, as well as the amount of calories and protein you are taking in. Many of the apps available have common brands and restaurants in their tracking system, so it is fairly easy to find what you ate! You do not need to record your food intake every day, especially since protein pacing does not focus on counting calories. Of course, food tracking is not required for this program. It's really for self-discovery. For example, you might think you are eating the same amount of food, but may actually be eating fewer calories that you did before you started protein pacing, or find that you are snacking less.

Another important thing to remember is hydration. Drinking more water, especially at meal times, can lead to feelings of fullness and help reduce hunger. Try to increase water intake in general, especially for those who do not typically drink a lot of water. Something I always found very interesting is that thirst can get mistaken for hunger, which can lead us to eat more when our bodies are not actually looking for more food! If you are trying to lose weight and are not normally a big water drinker, I would suggest drinking a glass of water first if you think that you are feeling hungry. If you still feel hungry after drinking, then definitely eat something. However, if you were actually thirsty and your body was misinterpreting the thirst signals, then you should no longer feel any sensation of hunger.

Each of us has different needs for fluid, and there really isn't a standard amount that is appropriate for everyone. It should be a goal to increase your fluid intake while you are protein pacing, especially if you are working out, as well. The best way to tell if you are hydrated enough is to look at the color of your urine. It should be a light yellow, like apple juice. If it is a color like dark amber, you need to drink more, as you are likely dehydrated. However, there are some medications that may change the color of your urine, and in these cases, it would not be an appropriate way to measure your hydration status.

Lastly, you'll soon learn that protein powder can get a little clumpy if it is not mixed right. I learned this because I made the mistake of thinking that I could just add the protein powder into a water bottle and shake it up. While it was not awful, there were some very noticeable clumps in the supplement as I was drinking it. That's not to say that you need to mix the whey protein and water in a blender. No one has time to clean a blender multiple times a day, and honestly, that would have been a deal breaker for me. Instead, I picked up a few blending bottles, and that made a world of difference. They are about the size of a regular reusable water bottle, but they are designed especially for mixing powdered supplements. Most come with either some type of ball or whisk inside, or they have a mesh layer that helps blend the powder better and break up any clumps. Plus, they are super easy to clean. You can find them at common retail stores, and they are not too expensive: My two bottles were less than $20 total after tax.

CHAPTER 9

SHOPPING FOR PROTEIN PACING

Now that you are ready to start protein pacing, the next step is to purchase a whey protein supplement, which will be used with any of the meal plan options discussed in Chapter 8. It can be confusing to know what to shop for, as there are different types of whey protein available. This chapter addresses the different types of whey protein supplements and what they mean. For those who are allergic to milk proteins or who prefer vegetable proteins, I have included information on other protein sources. Later in the chapter, I'll also talk about healthy fats, oils, and grains that you can incorporate into your protein pacing diet.

Whey Proteins

Whey is the liquid part of milk that remains after the cheese-making process. These leftover whey proteins are further separated using various processes. This will end up producing a few different forms of whey protein supplements; typically, there are three different types of whey protein available for purchase at most health food stores. These are whey protein concentrate, whey protein isolate, and hydrolyzed whey protein (whey protein hydrolysate). Although they are each technically a form of whey, they are actually pretty different!

As I mentioned earlier, whey protein is typically the preferred protein supplement due to its amino acid profile and how quickly it is absorbed into the bloodstream. Whey protein contains a lot of the essential amino acids, as well as something called branched chain amino acids, which are necessary in protein synthesis and may help in exercise performance (more on page 90). Because of these factors, whey is well-known as a protein with high biological value. Whey also has other vitamins and minerals, and is very commonly used in the food industry as an additive.

The type of whey protein that you choose will depend on your own personal goals and preferences. If you aren't sure which product to buy, you can stop by a specialty nutrition or supplement store and ask for assistance. However, most of the studies showed success with whey protein isolate, so this would be recommended if you do not have lactose intolerance.

One thing that stands out is the amount of protein between different types of whey, and how much lactose they contain. If you have a whey protein blend that has a much lower amount of protein grams per serving, you may not see much benefit from taking it. Whey protein concentrate is also more likely to affect someone with a lactose intolerance.

Whey protein concentrate. Whey protein concentrate is one of the cheaper forms of whey protein. Although it is still fairly low fat, it is higher in fat than whey protein isolate. Whey protein concentrate can contain anywhere from 30 to 80 percent protein, but many supplements available will have 70 to 80 percent protein. Some people prefer whey protein concentrate because it contains some compounds that are not found in whey protein isolate. For example, whey concentrates have higher levels of some growth factor hormones, and contain some carbohydrates. While these are not necessarily reasons to avoid whey protein concentrate, they may not be as well tolerated and do have slightly less protein than whey protein isolates. While product cost depends on the brand and the amount of servings, whey protein concentrate is cheaper than the isolate and hydrolyzed forms.

Whey protein isolate. Whey protein isolates are more highly processed, resulting in a purer product. Whey protein isolates are made up of at least 90 percent protein, but can contain as much as 96 percent protein. There are fewer other compounds in whey protein isolates, meaning that these supplements contain fewer fats and lactose. This would be a much better option for someone who has lactose intolerance. However, with the additional processing, whey protein isolates may have a breakdown to their structure, which could make them less effective than advertised. Whey protein isolates are more expensive than concentrates due to the extra processing.

Hydrolyzed whey protein (whey protein hydrolysate). Hydrolyzed whey protein is a product where the protein has been broken down into smaller protein parts. It contains around 90 percent protein. In other words, you can consider it pre-digested, meaning the amino acids will be available for use even sooner. Hydrolyzed whey protein is popular because it is thought to be absorbed faster since it is already pre-digested.

Hydrolyzed whey proteins are more expensive than whey protein concentrates, although the price is comparable to isolates.

Other Protein Supplements

If whey doesn't work for you or if you prefer to avoid animal products, there are a ton of different options available on the market that can be taken by themselves or in combination.

Branched chain amino acids (BCAAs). BCAAs are extremely popular among workout supplements. Not only do they help build new muscle, but they may help reduce the chance of protein and muscle breakdown during intense exercise. However, BCAA supplements only contain the three branched chain amino acids. This type of product has a specific use and is not meant to be a complete protein supplement. BCAAs would usually only be consumed right before, during, or immediately after a workout.

Brown rice protein. On its own, brown rice protein is not considered a complete protein because it does not contain all the essential amino acids. Brown rice protein is frequently mixed with another type of plant protein, such as quinoa, to make it a complete protein. This type of supplement mixes well with smoothies and often contains a small amount of fiber. Brown rice protein is vegetarian and vegan-friendly, and does not contain lactose. It can also be a good choice for someone with a lot of food allergies or sensitivities (always be sure to check ingredient labels!). However, it is considered to be inferior when it comes to muscle building and recovery, especially when compared to whey protein.

Shopping for Protein Pacing

Casein protein. Casein is the major part of protein that is found in cow's milk. It is another complete protein and contains calcium and phosphorus. When casein protein enters the stomach, it forms something that looks like a clot, which slows down how quickly it will leave the stomach. Since it will leave the stomach more slowly, it will also enter your bloodstream over a longer period. Casein protein is a popular option because it will provide amino acids over the course of a few hours, as opposed to whey, which is rapidly digested. This means that amino acids will be available to the muscles over a longer period than with whey. However, as noted on page 17, whey has a higher biological value than casein, and casein can be problematic for those with lactose intolerance.

Egg protein. Eggs are very well-known for being an excellent protein source. This type of protein is usually made from egg whites and is a source of protein with a high biological value. There is not as much available research on egg protein as compared to some of the other protein types. I would suggest it for those who prefer animal-based proteins but have milk allergies.

Hemp protein. Hemp protein is another good plant protein source, although it is not a complete protein. It is pretty easily digested, and has the benefit of containing omega 3 fatty acids. Hemp protein also provides BCAAs. Although hemp is typically thought of as being related to marijuana, it contains minimal amounts of THC (the effective substance in marijuana), and you cannot get high from it.

Mixed plant proteins. Mixed plant proteins can refer to any combination of plant-based proteins, and can provide an excellent source of protein to the diet. Some common plant proteins are peas, legumes, and hemp. Two or more proteins are mixed together in these products to provide a complete protein source. Since they are from multiple plant sources, these protein powders will often contain more fiber, which is usually well tolerated. However, this can slow digestion, so it may not be ideal for someone looking for a rapid source of amino acids. I strongly encourage anyone buying a mixed plant protein to read the product label to see exactly what you are purchasing, in case you have any allergies or food sensitivities.

Pea protein. Pea protein has become more popular in recent years, especially among vegetarians and vegans. It is made from the split yellow pea. Pea protein is also a good source of BCAAs. It can help improve satiety, and research has shown that it can help aid in muscle growth, as well.

Soy protein. Soy protein is the most common vegetable protein source. Soy products are used as a dietary staple in many Asian countries. It is very popular among people who are looking for a non-animal protein supplement, is considered a complete protein, and contains a lot of BCAAs. Most supplements will contain soy protein isolates, which contain greater than 90 percent protein. They are easily digested and mix well into foods and beverages. While soy protein did not show as much of a benefit as whey protein did in the study reviewed on page 31, it is still a great alternative for those looking to avoid animal products or for those who cannot tolerate whey.

Texturized vegetable protein (TVP). Although not a protein powder, this food product derives from soy flour. TVP can be an excellent addition to the diet, especially for vegetarians. It is a complete protein and can be made into alternative meat products (such as vegetarian burgers and hotdogs) or used on its own in recipes. It is a low-calorie and low-fat source of protein that is safe for people with milk or egg allergies. Anyone with a sensitivity or allergy to soy should avoid this product. Although TVP may look odd, it does not have a significant taste and will absorb the flavors of whatever you are cooking. I have included recipes using TVP in Chapter 10.

Fats and Oils

In many cases, you can be flexible about what type of oil you use for cooking. However, you need to be careful of recipes that involve heat. Olive oil has a reputation for being a very healthy type of oil, which it is, but it is not one you should be using with high heat, as high temperatures can cause it to break down. Not only can this change the taste of your food, but it can also be dangerous, as this can create free radicals. Free radicals are highly reactive, and can cause a chain reaction leading to cell damage.

Here, I've reviewed different types of cooking oils as well as what temperatures they are appropriate for. When I refer to the term smoke point, not only does that mean that the oil will start to smoke, but it also means that the oil will start to change chemically. Different variations of the types of oil (such as refined or unrefined) may alter the smoke point slightly. When using fats and oils, note the serving sizes, as these do have a lot of calories.

Avocado oil. Avocado oil is great for cooking because it can handle high heats very well. Unrefined versions of the oil are safe at temperatures up to 375°F to 400°F, and refined avocado oil has a smoke point of 520°F. I personally use avocado oil a lot since it is high in monounsaturated fats and I don't need to worry about how hot the food is getting. It is good for stir frying foods and searing.

Canola oil. Canola oil is a very multipurpose, mostly monounsaturated fat. Its smoke point is between 400°F and 425°F, and it is used in a variety of cooking methods.

Flaxseed oil. This type of oil is derived from flaxseeds and is mostly made up of polyunsaturated fats. One thing to note about flaxseed oil is that it has a low smoke point and is not a good choice for cooking. I would advise keeping flaxseed oil refrigerated and adding it to foods that are either served cold or have been previously cooked. The smoke point for flaxseed oil is only around 225°F.

Grapeseed oil. Grapeseed oil is widely used due to the very light taste. It is extracted from grape seeds that are left over from wine making and is high in omega-6 fatty acids. Its smoke point is about 420°F.

Olive oil. Olive oil is mostly made up of monounsaturated fats. The smoke point of olive oil depends on what type you buy. Extra virgin olive oil has a smoke point between 325°F and 375°F, while virgin and refined olive oils can handle slightly higher heat.

Peanut oil. Since peanut oil is derived from nuts, it should be avoided by anyone with an allergy. Half of the oil is made up of monounsaturated fats, while another third is polyunsaturated fats. Peanut oil can handle very high heats and is even good for deep frying, as it has a smoke point of around 450°F. Peanut oil is commonly used for frying and salad dressings.

Sesame oil. The smoke point of sesame oil varies between 350°F and 450°F, depending on the type you purchase. If you want to use sesame oil at a higher temperature, make sure you pick one that has been refined. Aside from being a good source of both polyunsaturated and monounsaturated fats, sesame oil is widely used in skin care items due to its high level of natural antioxidants.

Sunflower oil. Sunflower oil is another oil that is excellent for frying, with a smoke point of 440°F. It has a very mild flavor and color. Sunflower oil is derived from pressed sunflower seeds, and contains both monounsaturated and polyunsaturated fats.

Walnut oil. Walnut oil can be an excellent source of omega-3 fatty acids. It has a delicious nutty flavor that can be a great addition to recipes. Unrefined walnut oil has a low smoke point of 320°F and should not be used for cooking, but I highly recommend trying it on a salad. However, if you find a refined version, it can handle temperatures up to 400°F. Walnut oil is more perishable than other oil types, so be careful to check the expiration date. You may want to store this type of oil in the refrigerator.

High-Protein Grains and Grain Substitutes

Typical dietary staples like rice and pasta do contain some protein, but there are other grain varieties that have a much higher protein content. One way that you can increase the protein in your diet is to choose more of these high-protein whole grains. A grain is considered a whole grain if it contains all the original parts (the bran, the germ, and the endosperm). In comparison, a refined grain has been processed and stripped so that it only contains the endosperm. Be careful when you are buying grains to try to avoid pearled varieties, if possible. Pearled grains have gone through processing that allows for a faster cooking time. Since the bran has been removed, these grains have less fiber and can no longer be called a whole grain; however, pearling will not affect the protein content.

The higher protein grains I discuss here are not going to provide 20 grams of protein per serving (unless you eat multiple servings). However, choosing these higher protein and higher fiber grain products will still provide an additional nutritional benefit. I like to swap out more traditional food items for these grains to sneak in extra protein without much notice. I often will bring them as side dishes to parties, which can be a great conversation starter. I have found that most people are willing to try these grains that are unfamiliar to them, especially considering they look delicious! Plus, a lot of these grain foods are an easy substitute for more standard meal items, and they can all be eaten on their own. Some of them can be more expensive, but prices can be reasonable if you buy them in bulk. I like to make a batch of these on Sundays and incorporate them into different meals during the week to save myself time, as they can last well for a few days once they are prepared. If you have a hard time locating any of them, you can try ethnic specialty stores, or even consider ordering them online to make things easier.

The other benefit of adding more whole grains to your diet is they can help reduce the risk of chronic diseases, such as obesity, diabetes, heart disease, and certain types of cancer, since they contain higher amounts of fiber and more vitamins and minerals. So really, swapping out some of your normal food items should be a very logical choice.

Amaranth. Amaranth is a gluten-free grain that was a major food staple for the Aztecs. The flavor has been described as distinct, earthy, and nutty. It is an excellent source of manganese, and contains magnesium, iron, vitamin B6, folate, selenium, and zinc. It can be used on its own as a side dish, made into a hot breakfast cereal, or used to make breads and other baked goods.

One cup of cooked amaranth contains 250 calories, 5 grams of fiber, and 9 grams of protein.

Barley. Barley is a great source of fiber and is a higher protein grain product. Barley also contributes to your daily intake of potassium, vitamin B6, folate, manganese, and selenium. The type of fiber found in barley can help lower your LDL, or bad cholesterol, levels. It is commonly used in cereal products, but is also great on its own. Barley has a heartier texture than something like rice or pasta would. It is a chewier grain product, and does not get soft or mushy when cooking.

One cup of cooked barley contains about 190 calories, 6 grams of fiber, and 4 grams of protein.

Buckwheat. Buckwheat can be confusing as it is not technically wheat, nor is it a grain. It comes from seeds, which makes it gluten free. Buckwheat is a common ingredient in gluten-free products, and it is very popular among people who follow raw food diets. When buckwheat is toasted, it is referred to as kasha, which is commonly used in Central and Eastern Europe. Buckwheat is a source of magnesium, vitamin B6, and iron.

One cup of cooked buckwheat contains around 155 calories, 4.5 grams of fiber, and almost 6 grams of protein.

Bulgur. Bulgur is a food that we typically see in Middle Eastern cuisine. It is most commonly seen in tabbouleh salad, but can be a great substitute for rice as a side dish. It provides iron, vitamin B6, and magnesium.

One cup of cooked bulgur contains 150 calories, 8 grams of fiber, and 6 grams of protein.

Chia. Chia is technically a type of seed, and you probably would not consume this on its own. Chia seeds provide a lot of nutrition, contributing omega-3 fatty acids, calcium, manganese, magnesium, and phosphorus. Chia seeds are great mixed into hot cereals and smoothies. One interesting thing about chia seeds is that when they are soaked in liquid, they become gelatinous, and can be used to make puddings (find a recipe on page 124). While this is one of the lower protein foods on this list, I have included it due to the number of other health benefits that chia provides.

One tablespoon of chia seeds contains about 70 calories, 5 grams of fiber, and 2½ grams of protein.

Farro. Farro is one of my favorite grains. It is a whole grain that is a type of wheat. It has a mild, slightly nutty flavor and a chewier texture than rice (like barley). It is a good source of iron. Pre-soaking the farro can cut down on the cooking time, which normally takes up to 40 minutes. Ideally, it should be soaked overnight, but if that is not possible, a few hours will still make a difference in the total cooking time.

One cup of cooked farro contains 200 calories, 7 grams of fiber, and 8 grams of protein.

Freekeh. Freekeh is young green wheat that is a healthy, whole grain food. It is usually sold cracked, which cuts down on the total cooking time. It is a great source of selenium, potassium, zinc, and magnesium, in addition to providing protein and fiber.

One cup of cooked freekeh contains around 260 calories, 4 grams of fiber, and 8 grams of protein.

Kamut. Another name for kamut is Khorasan wheat, and it is a type of ancient grain. Ancient grains are types of grains and cereals that have changed very little over hundreds of years, as opposed to a product like corn. Kamut is not as chewy as some of the other grains, and does not have much of a taste. This makes it ideal as a base for recipes that may have other strong flavors.

One cup of cooked kamut contains 250 calories, less than 2 grams of fat, 7 grams of fiber, and 11 grams of protein.

Lentils. Lentils are considered part of the legume family and are not technically grains. The most common lentils you will see are the brown and green types, as they hold their shape best even after cooking. Lentils provide a number of micronutrients, including molybdenum, folate, copper, phosphorus, manganese, iron, vitamin B1, pantothenic acid, and zinc.

One cup of cooked lentils contains 230 calories, less than 1 gram of fat, 16 grams of fiber, and 18 grams of protein.

Quinoa. One of the most mispronounced foods I've ever heard, this is actually said KEEN-wah. Technically, quinoa is not classified as a grain, but nutritionally it is used as one. Quinoa is in the amaranth family and it has been cultivated for thousands of years. Not only is it gluten free, but it is a complete protein that contains all the essential amino acids. It contains magnesium, manganese, folate, phosphorus, copper, iron, and zinc. One interesting thing about quinoa is that it naturally has a coating that acts as an insecticide, which is easily rinsed off. Quinoa is very easy to incorporate into your diet, and it is commonly used as a substitute for rice. It can also be used in baking, as a breakfast grain, in salads, and to make veggie burgers.

One cup of cooked quinoa contains 225 calories, 5 grams of fiber, and 8 grams of protein.

Spelt. Spelt is a type of wheat that has been used since 5,000 BC. It is another whole grain food that can be substituted in many recipes, and the flour is commonly used to make breads. It provides manganese, phosphorus, vitamin B3, magnesium, iron, and zinc.

One cup of cooked spelt contains about 250 calories, 7 grams of fiber, and 10 grams of protein.

Teff. Teff is a gluten-free whole grain that originated in Africa. It is quickly becoming more mainstream, as it is looked at as one of the ancient grains. Unlike many other whole grains, it does not contain gluten. Teff provides more calcium than many other grain products, in addition to being a good source of iron, magnesium, phosphorus, manganese, and copper.

One cup cooked teff contains 255 calories, 7 grams of fiber, and almost 10 grams of protein.

Wheat berries. Wheat berries are the whole, uncracked version of wheat that are technically seeds, not berries. They are not processed, meaning that they are not stripped of their nutritional value. Wheat berries are a good source of magnesium, in addition to containing folate, many B vitamins, and vitamin E.

One cup of cooked wheat berries contains 300 calories, 8 grams of fiber, and 12 grams of protein.

CHAPTER 10

RECIPES

Although it is not necessary to change your normal diet when you start protein pacing, making some swaps in your diet to include healthier options can help you lose weight faster. Some of these recipes may be very similar to ones you normally eat and could be easy to substitute. Other recipes may be a bit more adventurous and fun to try. Some of the recipes are excellent sources of high biological value protein, which will maximize the benefits of increasing your protein intake. Other recipes use whey protein as one of the ingredients to provide increased protein. I have included a variety of food types, different flavor backgrounds, and preparation methods so that the recipes may be helpful to you depending on your lifestyle, preferences, and time constraints.

Purple People Eater Smoothie

MAKES: 1 (1½-cup) serving
COOK TIME: 1 minute

1 scoop preferred protein powder

¼ cup frozen blueberries

⅛ cup rolled oats

1 tablespoon all-natural peanut butter

1 cup cold water

Add all ingredients into blender and blend on high for 30 seconds. Pour into a cup and serve chilled.

EspressPro Smoothie

MAKES: 1 (2-cup) serving
COOK TIME: 1 minute

1 scoop preferred protein powder

10 teaspoons fat-free or low-fat plain Greek yogurt

½ banana

2 tablespoons brewed espresso

1 cup unsweetened cashew or almond milk

1 cup ice

Use a blender to blend all ingredients together on medium, and serve chilled.

Monkey's Lunch Smoothie

MAKES: 1 (2-cup) serving

COOK TIME: 1 minute

1 scoop preferred protein powder

¼ cup dried oats

½ banana

½ cup strawberries

1 tablespoon all-natural peanut butter

1 cup ice cubes

1 cup water

Use a blender to blend all ingredients on high until smooth.

Protein Acai-Fruit Bowl

In this recipe, the fruit is added as a topping. However, if you prefer a more traditional acai bowl, blend the fruit with the protein powder and Greek yogurt.

MAKES: 1 (1¼-cup) serving

COOK TIME: 10 minutes

½ scoop preferred protein powder

½ cup fat-free or low-fat plain Greek yogurt

4 ounces acai or berries of choice

3 tablespoons nuts of choice

1 tablespoon chia seeds

1 tablespoon shredded coconut

1. Blend Greek yogurt and protein powder together in a blender or food processor.

2. Top with fruit, nuts, chia seeds, and shredded coconut.

Peanut Butter and Jelly Ice Cream Smoothie

High-protein ice cream has gained a lot of popularity recently because these products are often much lower in calories compared to traditional ice cream, have less sugar, and contain a lot more protein. I also used powdered peanut butter in this recipe, because it easily mixes into recipes and has fewer calories than the original version. Where 2 tablespoons of peanut butter would have almost 200 calories and 16 grams of fat, 2 tablespoons of the powdered version have around 45 calories and 1½ grams of fat. Feel free to use 1 tablespoon all-natural peanut butter in this recipe for a heartier serving.

If you prefer a thinner smoothie, you can add more almond milk to the recipe as needed. For a thicker smoothie, freeze the strawberries before blending. Soy milk can be substituted for almond, and strawberry ice cream can be used for a fruitier smoothie.

MAKES: 2 (1-cup) servings

COOK TIME: 1 minute

1 cup high-protein vanilla ice cream

½ scoop preferred vanilla-flavored protein powder

1 cup unsweetened almond milk

2 tablespoons powdered peanut butter

2 tablespoons strawberry preserves

½ cup strawberries

1 cup ice

Use a blender to combine all ingredients. Enjoy!

Strawberry Banana High-Protein Shake

This shake can easily be modified to include your favorite fruits. Substitute out the strawberries for blueberries or raspberries, or throw in a handful of spinach for some extra iron.

MAKES: 1 (1½-cup) serving

COOK TIME: 1 minute

1 plus ½ teaspoons chia seeds

½ cup soy milk, plus more as needed

½ cup orange juice

½ frozen banana

4 frozen strawberries

1 scoop whey protein powder

1 teaspoon coconut oil

Combine all ingredients in a blender and blend until smooth. Add additional soy milk as needed if shake is too thick.

High-Protein Muffins

Muffins are a popular breakfast choice, but can be a nightmare for anyone who is trying to lose weight. Some of the worst ones contain cream cheese and streusel toppings, and may contain over 500 calories. High-protein muffins are a great substitution and can help take care of any muffin craving that you might have.

These muffins are made with whey protein and do not contain any flour, which makes them gluten free. Each muffin contains around 25 grams of protein. For high-protein chocolate chip muffins, use chocolate protein powder and mix in ¼ cup of dark chocolate chips to the batter before pouring in the muffin tin.

MAKES: 4 muffins

COOK TIME: 20 minutes

½ ripe medium banana

1 egg

½ teaspoon baking soda

2 tablespoons milk

5 tablespoons preferred protein powder

1. Preheat oven to 350°F.

2. Using a fork, mash banana well in a large bowl.

3. In a small bowl, whisk the egg. Add egg to the mashed banana.

4. Add baking soda, milk, and whey protein to liquid mixture.

5. In a nonstick muffin pan, fill up four muffin spots to about ¾ of the way full. If you do not have a nonstick muffin pan, coat each muffin spot with a small amount of cooking spray.

Recipes

6. Bake muffins at 350°F for 20 minutes.

7. Let muffins cool for about 30 minutes before removing them from the muffin pan. Serve and enjoy.

Banana Oatmeal Protein Muffins

These muffins are delicious with mix-ins like chocolate chips or slivered almonds.

MAKES: 12 muffins

COOK TIME: 20 minutes

coconut oil spray, for greasing tray

2 scoops preferred protein powder

2 whole eggs

2 cups rolled oats

2 bananas

1 cup fat-free or low-fat plain Greek yogurt

⅓ cup raw honey

1 teaspoon vanilla extract

½ teaspoon baking soda

1½ teaspoons baking powder

optional mix-ins

1. Preheat oven to 400°F.

2. Spray muffin pan with coconut oil.

3. Mix all ingredients together in a medium bowl. Pour mixture into muffin tray.

4. Bake for 20 minutes. Let muffins cool before eating.

Fat-Free Pumpkin Pancakes

Feel free to divide the batter to enjoy more delicious pancakes. Serve with your favorite whipped topping and pancake syrup.

MAKES: 1 large pancake

COOK TIME: 6 minutes

½ scoop preferred protein powder

4 large egg whites

1 tablespoon pumpkin puree

1 teaspoon vanilla

1 teaspoon baking powder

coconut oil spray, for greasing pan

1. Mix protein powder, egg whites, pumpkin puree, vanilla, and baking powder in a blender, and blend until smooth.

2. Heat a nonstick pan over medium heat. Spray with coconut oil.

3. Add mixture to pan and cook each side for 2 to 3 minutes, or until they are both golden brown.

Low-Carb Pancakes

Enjoy with 1 teaspoon of melted coconut oil and a drizzle of pancake syrup.

MAKES: 1 large pancake

COOK TIME: 6 minutes

½ scoop preferred protein powder

4 large egg whites

1 teaspoon cinnamon

coconut oil spray, for greasing pan

1. Mix protein powder, egg whites, and cinnamon in a blender, and blend until smooth.

2. Heat a nonstick pan over medium heat. Spray with coconut oil.

3. Add mixture to pan and cook each side for 2 to 3 minutes, or until they are both golden brown.

Two-Ingredient Banana Pancakes

This recipe only has two ingredients that are usually found in most people's homes: eggs and bananas. I think they taste great plain, but if you want additional flavor, you can top them with a tablespoon of honey, a drizzle of agave syrup, melted peanut butter, or a small pat of butter.

MAKES: 3 to 4 small pancakes; 1 serving

COOK TIME: 10 minutes

　　1 small ripe banana
　　1 whole egg
　　2 egg whites

1. Using a fork, mash the banana in a medium bowl until it is as broken up as possible.

2. Add in the whole egg and egg whites. Mix together until the batter looks even throughout.

3. Heat a large greased frying pan over medium heat.

4. Pour the batter slowly into the frying pan until you've made a pancake about 2 inches in diameter. Repeat with the rest of the batter to make about 4 pancakes.

5. Carefully flip each pancake when it browns, 2 to 3 minutes.

Two-Ingredient Oatmeal Pancakes: Replace the banana with ½ cup rolled oats. Blend oats in a blender or food processor until they become a fine powder. Transfer to a medium bowl and follow steps 2 through 5 above.

High-Protein Overnight Oats

Overnight oats is one of my favorite ways to prepare oatmeal. Not only are they extremely easy to make, but they can also save you a lot of time in the morning, since you prepare everything the night before! You can add in other fruits or other toppings as you desire, such as chopped nuts, berries, or shredded coconut. The oatmeal and any added fruit can be a good source of dietary fiber. You can also add almond or peanut butter in the blender with the other ingredients for a serving of healthy fat. This recipe makes one serving of oats.

MAKES: 1 (1½-cup) serving

COOK TIME: 1 minute

½ cup fat-free or low-fat plain Greek yogurt

½ cup water

1 scoop preferred protein powder

1 teaspoon vanilla extract

¾ cup rolled oats

1. Use a blender to combine Greek yogurt, water, protein powder, and vanilla.

2. Stir mixture into rolled oats and blend well with a spoon.

3. Transfer to a container with a lid and refrigerate overnight. Serve chilled.

Apple Cinnamon Overnight Oats

MAKES: 1 (1-cup) serving

COOK TIME: 1 minute

½ scoop preferred protein powder

½ cup fat-free or low-fat plain Greek yogurt

¼ cup rolled oats

½ medium green apple, cubed

1 tablespoon coconut oil

1 teaspoon vanilla extract

½ teaspoon nutmeg

2 tablespoons sugar-free caramel sauce

1 tablespoon cinnamon

1. Mix all ingredients together in a medium bowl.

2. Transfer to a container with a lid and refrigerate overnight. Serve chilled.

Pumpkin Spice Latte Overnight Oats: In the fall, try this seasonal variation using 1 scoop preferred vanilla protein powder, ¼ cup oats, ⅓ cup black coffee, 1 tablespoon fat-free or low-fat plain Greek yogurt, 1 tablespoon pumpkin puree,1 teaspoon cinnamon, and 1 teaspoon pumpkin spice blend.

Tomato and Kale Egg-White Quiche

Quiche is one of my favorite brunch foods, and I'll often make it for company. It's delicious and has a ton of flavor. It is also appropriate for anyone following a vegetarian diet. You can use a liquid egg white product if you do not want to waste the egg yolks. If you are using a container of liquid egg whites, follow the guidelines on the carton for how to substitute.

MAKES: 1 (9-inch) quiche; 8 servings

COOK TIME: 45 minutes

1 teaspoon dried basil or fresh chopped basil	1½ cups chopped kale, stems removed
½ teaspoon dried thyme	15 to 16 large egg whites
¼ teaspoon chili powder	1 medium tomato, chopped
¼ teaspoon ground paprika	¼ cup shredded mozzarella or 2 ounces fresh mozzarella, sliced thinly
½ teaspoon ground turmeric	

1. Preheat oven to 325°F. Use cooking spray to coat a 9-inch round baking pan.

2. Mix spices together and set aside.

3. In a large bowl, massage each piece of kale until it starts to soften and looks brighter green. This should take 3 to 5 minutes.

4. In another large bowl, whisk the egg whites until they turn frothy. Then add spices and whisk again.

5. Spread the tomato and kale over the bottom of the baking pan. Evenly spread the cheese on top.

6. Gently pour the egg whites on top of the vegetables and cheese so as not to displace the bottom ingredients.

7. Bake at 325°F for 40 to 45 minutes. To test doneness, stick a toothpick into the center of the quiche; it should come out clean.

8. Allow quiche to cool for 5 to 10 minutes prior to serving.

Homemade Chocolate Protein Bars

Protein bars can be a great snack or meal replacement, especially when you are running around and don't have time to sit down for a real meal. The bad thing about protein bars is that they can be really expensive, or have a lot of ingredients and you aren't sure what they are or if they are even good for you. In this case, there are only 7 ingredients, and they are all things that you can easily recognize!

If you do not want to add chocolate chips or prefer other flavors, you can substitute with any type of chopped nuts, peanut butter chips, coconut flakes, or dried fruit in the same proportion.

MAKES: 8 (1-bar) servings

COOK TIME: 1 hour refrigeration

1 cup almond butter

3 tablespoons unsweetened almond milk

¼ cup agave syrup

1 tablespoon cocoa powder

4 scoops preferred chocolate protein powder

½ cup rolled oats

¼ cup chocolate chips (optional)

1. Line an 8 x 8-inch baking pan with waxed paper and set aside.

2. Mix together almond butter, almond milk, and agave syrup in a medium bowl. Stir until well blended.

3. Add in cocoa powder, protein powder, and rolled oats. Mix well until ingredients are well blended and have formed a dough.

4. Work the chocolate chips into the dough.

5. Press the dough evenly into the baking pan. Refrigerate for at least 1 hour.

6. Remove from refrigerator and cut into 8 equal-sized bars. Store bars in refrigerator or freezer.

Chocolate Chip High-Protein Zucchini Bread

Zucchini bread is one of my favorite things to bake, but it is a very high carbohydrate food that does not provide much protein. This alternative recipe requires the addition of a protein powder of your choice. It also contains fiber, which aids in gut health. I use plain or vanilla-flavored whey protein powder in this recipe, but you can substitute plant-based protein powders. Depending on the flavor of the protein powder that you choose, you can leave out the cocoa powder and the chocolate. You can choose to substitute almond butter for peanut butter, which is also delicious.

MAKES: 12 (1-slice) servings

COOK TIME: 1 hour

¾ cup all-natural peanut butter

¼ cup maple syrup

2 large eggs, lightly whisked, or ½ cup egg substitute

1 tablespoon vanilla extract

1 cup shredded zucchini

2 scoops preferred protein powder

1 teaspoon baking soda

1 tablespoon cocoa powder (optional)

½ cup plus 1 tablespoon chocolate chips, divided (optional)

1. Preheat oven to 350°F and grease an 8 x 4-inch loaf pan.

2. In a large bowl, mix together peanut butter, maple syrup, eggs, and vanilla until well blended.

3. Add zucchini into liquid mixture and stir well.

4. In a small bowl, whisk together protein powder, baking soda, and cocoa powder. Combine well, and then add to wet ingredients. Mix gently.

5. Mix ½ cup of chocolate chips into batter.

6. Pour the batter into the greased loaf pan and make sure the mixture is spread evenly throughout pan.

7. Sprinkle the top of the mixture with the remaining 1 table-spoon of chocolate chips.

8. Bake at 350°F for 45 minutes. Check for doneness by inserting a toothpick into the center of the bread; it should come out clean.

9. Allow bread to cool on a wire rack for about 30 minutes prior to serving.

Mexican Frittata

Eggs are a great source of protein that can be eaten for any meal. Frittatas are an easy way to get in high-quality protein and vegetables, and can be reheated for later meals.

MAKES: 4 servings

COOK TIME: 25 minutes

½ tablespoon olive oil

2 scallions, finely chopped

1 red pepper, chopped

3 large eggs

1 teaspoon dried cilantro

salt and pepper, to taste

¼ cup shredded pepper jack cheese

1. Preheat oven to 425°F.

2. Add olive oil to an 8" oven-safe skillet and heat over medium heat.

3. When oil is heated, add scallions and red pepper. Cook until soft, about 5 minutes.

4. Whisk the eggs in a medium bowl. Add cilantro, salt, and pepper.

5. Add egg mixture to skillet. Cook for about 10 minutes, using a spatula to lift the edges so that any uncooked egg settles to the bottom of the pan.

6. Sprinkle cheese evenly over the top of the egg mixture. Then, move pan to the oven and bake about 10 minutes, until the frittata is puffy and golden.

7. Serve warm or at room temperature.

Chili Lime Roasted Chickpeas

Chickpeas, also known as garbanzo beans, are a great source of fiber and protein and make a healthy alternative to chips or pretzels. Typically, after I dry the chickpeas, I allow them to sit out for a little while and then I dry them again. Any excess moisture means they will not get crunchy when you are baking them. The oil I used can be substituted for a different heat-appropriate oil, though cooking times may vary slightly.

MAKES: About 3 (½-cup) servings

COOK TIME: 50 minutes

1 (15-ounce) can chickpeas

¼ cup sesame oil

1½ teaspoons chili powder

1½ teaspoons grated lime zest

1. Drain chickpeas using a colander and rinse well. Preheat the oven to 400°F.

2. Using paper towels, pat chickpeas. Allow to air dry for about 20 minutes. Repeat until dry.

3. Drizzle chickpeas lightly with sesame oil. Mix well to ensure that all of them are coated.

4. Sprinkle with chili powder and lime zest, and mix well so that all beans are covered.

5. Roast in the oven for approximately 30 minutes.

Chia Seed Pudding

For such a tiny seed, chia can provide many health benefits. It contributes omega-3 fatty acids, calcium, manganese, magnesium, and phosphorus. When I make chia seed pudding, I personally like to store it in baby food jars, as it is the perfect serving size. The texture is different from what you may be used to, but it is worth trying, as it can be such a delicious healthy treat! This recipe makes four servings.

MAKES: 4 (½-cup) servings

COOK TIME: 5 minutes, plus 5 hours refrigeration

2 cups coconut or almond milk

½ teaspoon pure vanilla extract

⅛ cup agave syrup

½ cup chia seeds

½ cup fresh berries

1. Mix coconut or almond milk, vanilla extract, and agave syrup together in a medium bowl.

2. Add chia seeds and whisk well to stir.

3. Gently pour chia seed mixture into individual containers or a single storage container, then cover.

4. Refrigerate overnight, or for at least 5 hours. For first 1 to 2 hours, stir mixture a few times so that the pudding has an even texture and consistency.

5. Top with fresh berries prior to serving.

Protein Pudding

MAKES: 1 (¾-cup) serving

COOK TIME: 1 minute

½ scoop preferred protein powder

½ cup fat-free or low-fat plain Greek yogurt

Mix ingredients well in a blender or food processor until smooth, and enjoy.

High-Protein Almond Butter Balls

This is one of my favorite recipes because it is so quick and easy to make. It also stores well in the freezer. They are meant to be snacks, but you can eat more than one for a quick, on-the-go breakfast. Each ball is one serving.

MAKES: 25 (1-inch) balls

COOK TIME: 3 hours

2 cups crunchy almond butter

2 tablespoons cocoa powder

2 scoops preferred protein powder

2 mashed ripe bananas

2 tablespoons flaxseeds

1. In a large bowl, mix together almond butter, cocoa, protein powder, bananas, and flaxseeds. Mix very well using a wooden spoon.

2. Roll mixture into balls that are about 1 inch in diameter.

3. Place balls in a container lined with parchment paper. Use additional parchment to separate layers so balls do not stick together.

4. Freeze protein balls for 2 to 3 hours before serving.

Healthy Pulled Pork

This recipe requires the use of a slow cooker, but total prepara-tion time is less than 10 minutes. This recipe works well for meal prep, and reheats well. Enjoy as a sandwich on a whole grain roll or served over quinoa and veggies.

MAKES: 6 (8-ounce) servings

COOK TIME: 6 hours

1 teaspoon ground paprika

1 teaspoon ground turmeric

1 teaspoon ground black pepper

½ teaspoon garlic powder

¼ teaspoon ground ginger

¼ teaspoon ground cinnamon

¼ cup olive oil

2½ pounds pork tenderloin

1½ cups chicken or vegetable stock

1. In a small bowl, mix all spices together. Add olive oil to spices and mix well.

2. Place the pork in slow cooker. Evenly pour spice mixture over pork.

3. Pour the chicken or vegetable stock on top of pork.

4. Cook for 6 hours on low setting.

5. After 6 hours, use two forks to pull the meat apart. It will fall apart easily.

Textured Vegetable Protein (TVP) Sloppy Joes

This is a fun option for anyone following a vegan or vegetarian diet, or for someone who just wants to limit how many animal products they are eating. TVP will be lower in fat than meat products, and contains no cholesterol. It also contains much less sodium than traditional Sloppy Joes would, depending on how much hot sauce you add. This recipe can be great for kids, but keep in mind that this recipe lives up to its name: It's a mess. I would recommend keeping plenty of napkins on hand.

Use your favorite variety of bell peppers and onion. When serving, choose a whole grain roll that contains fiber to add more nutrition.

MAKES: 6 (¾-cup) servings

COOK TIME: 45 minutes

avocado oil, for sautéing

2 medium bell peppers, diced

1 medium onion, diced

1 cup tomato sauce

2½ cups low-sodium vegetable broth

1 tablespoon chili powder

1 tablespoon soy sauce

hot sauce, to taste

1½ cups TVP, plus ½ cup more at a time, if needed

1 tablespoon arrowroot powder (optional)

salt and pepper, to taste

1. Heat avocado oil in a medium skillet over medium-high heat. Sauté peppers and onions until softened.

2. Reduce heat. Mix in tomato sauce and vegetable broth. Stir until well combined.

3. Once mixture is slowly bubbling, add chili powder, soy sauce, and desired amount of hot sauce.

4. Mix in TVP and stir well.

5. Allow to simmer for at least 15 minutes. Season with salt and pepper, to taste.

6. Remove skillet from heat. Mixture should thicken as it cools down. If it still appears too watery after cooling, add a small amount of arrowroot powder to thicken, or add more TVP and simmer for another 15 minutes.

Turkey Chili

Turkey chili is one of my favorite fall and winter recipes. I also will make it in the summer and throw it over some mixed greens for a healthy salad. Not only can it be prepared relatively quickly, but you can make it ahead of time and either refrigerate it or freeze it. And you can make it all in one pot, which saves a lot of time cleaning up!

Four ounces of 93-percent lean ground turkey has about 160 calories and 20 grams of protein. If purchasing canned beans, find a variety that has little or no added sodium (you can usually find brands that contain less than 100 milligrams per serving). Some brands add so much salt as a preservative that each can may have over a whole day's worth of sodium in it! You can also find a low-sodium chili seasoning mix if you prefer to use a premade packet and avoid dealing with all the spices.

MAKES: 6 (1-cup) servings

COOK TIME: 40 minutes

2 tablespoons ground cumin

1½ teaspoons ground paprika

1 teaspoon powdered dried onion

1 teaspoon dried basil

1 teaspoon ground turmeric

red chili powder, to taste

3 tablespoons avocado oil

1 pound 93-percent lean ground turkey

1 (15-ounce) can low-sodium black beans

1 (15-ounce) can low-sodium kidney beans

2 (6-ounce) cans tomato paste

1½ cups water

1. In a small bowl, mix all the spices together. Set aside.

2. Add the avocado oil to a large pot and place over medium heat.

3. Add the ground turkey to the heated pot and break into small pieces using a wooden spoon. Cook over medium heat until all the turkey meat has been cooked through (approximately 15 minutes).

4. Add black beans, kidney beans, tomato paste, and water. Mix until well blended. Keep over medium heat until chili begins to bubble.

5. Add spices and stir until well blended. Allow chili to return to a slow bubble.

6. Remove from heat and serve, or store for future meals.

Vegan Textured Vegetable Protein (TVP) Chili

While I do love my Turkey Chili (page 130), this is another version I frequently prepare. It is easy and stores well for later use. It's also great to make for potlucks or when cooking for large groups of people. Some people have actually not been able to tell that it is vegetarian, since it is so flavorful.

Feel free to add in additional vegetables as desired. I like to choose two different colored peppers for more color and different nutrients. You can also leave out the TVP if you want and make a plain vegetable chili, but that version will not have as much protein.

MAKES: 4 (¾-cup) servings

COOK TIME: 60 minutes

½ yellow onion, diced

2 bell peppers, diced

2 cloves garlic, diced

2 tablespoons olive oil

1 (15-ounce) can diced tomatoes, with juice

¼ cup vegetable broth

1–2 tablespoons chili powder, or to taste

½ teaspoon cayenne pepper, or to taste

1 (15-ounce) can black beans, drained

1 (15-ounce) can kidney beans, drained

½ cup TVP

salt and pepper, to taste

1. In a large skillet or sauté pan, sauté onion, peppers, and diced garlic in olive oil over medium heat for a few minutes until vegetables are soft.

2. To the skillet, add the diced tomatoes with juice, vegetable broth, chili powder, and cayenne pepper. Stir until well combined.

3. Decrease to medium-low heat and add black beans and kidney beans. Cook 15 to 20 minutes. The chili should be slowly bubbling. Stir occasionally to prevent chili from burning.

4. Add TVP and enough water to achieve desired thickness. Cook for at least 15 minutes.

5. Season with salt and pepper to taste. Serve.

Lentil Soup

I love lentils because they provide a great source of protein and fiber, as well as having several micronutrients. Lentil soup may not sound that interesting, but it can be the basis for a hearty meal. The combination of protein, fiber, and fluid tends to be extremely filling. I like to serve this recipe with warm pita bread for dipping. It is also delicious with French or Italian bread.

I find myself making this a lot in the winter, although you can definitely eat it all year round. This soup freezes well, so I often make it in larger batches. If you are doubling the recipe, do not double the spices. Use the original amount of seasoning and then add more to taste. If you double the spices, you may end up with an overpowering flavor.

MAKES: 4 (2-cup) servings

COOK TIME: 1 hour, 10 minutes

2 cups dried green lentils	1 (14-ounce) can crushed tomatoes
2 tablespoons olive oil	
1 medium yellow onion, diced	1½ quarts low-sodium vegetable broth
1 garlic clove, minced	½ teaspoon cumin
2 celery stalks, chopped	1½ teaspoon ground paprika
2 large carrots, chopped	salt and pepper, to taste
	3 pitas, each cut in half

1. Rinse lentils and drain well, then set aside.

2. Heat oil in a large pot over medium heat. Add onion and garlic and cook for 3 to 4 minutes.

3. Add in celery and carrots and cook for another 10 minutes. At this point, the vegetables should be softened, and the onion should start to caramelize.

4. Add in lentils, crushed tomatoes, vegetable broth, cumin, and paprika. Mix well. Add salt and pepper to taste.

5. Turn up heat slightly and bring soup to a simmer. Skim the surface of the soup when it develops a skin on top using a large metal spoon.

6. Turn the heat down to medium low. Cover soup and cook for about 40 minutes, until lentils are soft. If you prefer a thinner soup, add more broth, and stir well to incorporate.

7. Serve with warmed pita bread.

Asian Chicken Stir Fry

I love Asian stir fries, but when you order take out, you can end up with something loaded with calories, fat, and sodium. Homemade stir fries are a great meal idea year-round. One of the best things about stir fry recipes is that you can pack them with extra vegetables. The chicken in this recipe can easily be substituted with beef or tofu, or you can keep it to be made entirely out of vegetables (but you would need another protein source at the meal!). This recipe version uses quinoa instead of the traditional white rice for more protein and fiber, but you could easily swap in a different high-protein, high-fiber grain.

MAKES: 4 (2-cup) servings

COOK TIME: 1 hour, 20 minutes

2 cups quinoa

⅔ cup low-sodium soy sauce

¼ cup brown sugar

1 tablespoon corn starch

1 tablespoon minced fresh ginger

1 clove garlic, minced, or more to taste

3 boneless skinless chicken breasts, sliced into thin strips

2 tablespoons sesame oil, divided

1 red bell pepper, cut into thin strips

1 cup sugar snap peas

2 cups broccoli florets

1 cup thin sliced carrots

1 medium yellow onion, chopped

1. Prepare quinoa according to package directions.

2. In a small bowl, mix together soy sauce, brown sugar, and corn starch until well combined. Add the ginger and garlic into sauce and mix well.

3. Cover chicken strips with marinade and place in refrigerator for at least 15 minutes.

4. Add 1 tablespoon of the sesame oil in a large skillet or wok over medium-high heat. Add bell pepper strips, sugar snap peas, broccoli, carrots, and onion. Cook until vegetables are tender, about 5 minutes. Remove vegetables from the skillet and keep warm.

5. Remove the chicken strips from the marinade, but do not discard liquid.

6. Heat the remaining tablespoon of sesame oil in the skillet or wok over medium-high heat. Cook and stir chicken for 2 to 3 minutes on each side. The chicken should be mostly cooked but may still have a slightly pink center.

7. Add the rest of the marinade to skillet and stir well. Return the vegetables to the skillet and cook, stirring well, for 5 to 7 minutes, or until chicken is completely cooked through.

8. Serve over quinoa.

Spicy High-Protein Chicken Quinoa Soup with TVP

Making simple modifications can easily increase the nutritional value of a recipe. Homemade chicken noodle soup is one of my favorites, but it doesn't necessarily contain a good serving of protein. By swapping out noodles for quinoa and adding TVP, you increase the protein content for this hearty dish that eats more like a stew.

MAKES: 5 (2-cup) servings

COOK TIME: 40 minutes

1 tablespoon olive oil

1 medium onion, chopped

4 celery stalks, chopped

2 cups chopped carrots

⅓ teaspoon chili powder, or to taste

⅓ teaspoon powdered cayenne pepper, or to taste

1 cup quinoa

3 cups water

1 quart low-sodium chicken broth

1 cup TVP

2 cups chopped broccoli florets

2½ cups cooked, shredded white meat chicken

salt and pepper, to taste

1. Heat olive oil in a large pot over medium heat.

2. Add onion, celery, carrots, chili powder, and cayenne pepper. Cook for about 5 minutes, stirring regularly.

3. Add the quinoa, water, chicken broth, and TVP to the pot. Cook for 10 to 15 minutes, until the quinoa begins to soften.

4. Add broccoli and cook for another 5 minutes.

5. Add chicken and stir well. Add salt and pepper, to taste.

6. Remove from heat and serve.

High-Protein Chocolate Chip Almond Cookies

I like cookies as an occasional snack, but I'm always on the hunt for a healthier version. This recipe makes a moist, delicious cookie; protein powder makes it a higher protein, healthier treat. Use an unflavored variety to let the almond butter and chocolate chip flavors stand out. If you refrigerate your almond butter, take it out and let it get to room temperature. The almond butter can also be substituted with peanut or cashew butter. These cookies freeze well; I suggest defrosting them in the microwave for best taste.

MAKES: 12 cookies

COOK TIME: 25 minutes

2 very ripe medium bananas

2 scoops preferred protein powder

1 cup quick-cooking oats

2 tablespoons almond butter

2 tablespoons mini chocolate chips

1. Preheat oven to 350°F.

2. In a medium bowl, mash bananas with a fork until they are somewhat smooth.

3. Mix in protein powder, oats, and almond butter until smooth. The batter may be a little runny; that's OK.

4. Mix in the mini chocolate chips.

5. Line a baking sheet with waxed paper. Spoon 12 scoops of batter onto the sheet.

6. Bake cookies for 12 minutes. Cool for 5 minutes on a cooling rack before serving.

Peanut Butter Black Bean Brownies

I admit, when I first heard of black bean brownies, I thought they would be terrible. I've tried a few recipes that tasted too bean-y, or were dry and had no flavor. Since black beans are such a great source of nutrition, I knew I had to keep trying until I found a delicious black bean brownie recipe. I have given this to people without telling them it included black beans, and only one person suspected that they were made with "something healthy." One fantastic thing about these brownies is that the recipe does not contain eggs, so if you prefer them slightly undercooked, there is no risk of foodborne illness. If you have a peanut allergy, the peanut butter chips can be substituted with regular chocolate chips.

MAKES: 8 brownies

COOK TIME: 30 minutes

1 (15-ounce) can black beans

2 tablespoons cocoa powder

½ cup quick-cooking oats

¼ teaspoon salt

½ cup maple syrup

¼ cup coconut oil

2 teaspoons vanilla extract

½ teaspoon baking powder

⅔ cup peanut butter chips

1. Preheat oven to 350°F. Grease an 8 x 8-inch baking pan.

2. Add the black beans, cocoa powder, oats, salt, maple syrup, coconut oil, vanilla, and baking powder to a food processor. Run until mixture is completely smooth, with no lumps.

3. Add brownie batter to a large mixing bowl and mix in the peanut butter chips. Scoop mixture into the baking pan and press into an even layer.

Recipes

4. Cook brownies for 16 minutes.

5. Let brownies cool for about 1 hour prior to serving.

Healthy High-Protein Cheesecake

Cheesecake is an extremely popular dessert item that, unfortunately, is not so healthy. A small slice is OK once in a while, but portions can easily get out of control. Some cheesecakes served in chain restaurants contain over 1,500 calories in a single slice, not to mention the fat and sugar content!

This recipe is high-protein, low-carbohydrate, and delicious. For the crust, I have used cinnamon graham crackers and honey graham crackers, and both have come out delicious. You could use a chocolate or vanilla yogurt or protein powder in this recipe if you'd like to make a flavored version. Do not use a fat-free cream cheese. If you want additional toppings, you can always add crushed cookies, nuts, more graham crackers, etc., to the top of the cheesecake prior to baking, but keep in mind that any extra toppings will add more calories.

MAKES: 1 cheesecake; 8 servings

COOK TIME: 1 hour, 30 minutes

8 ounces light cream cheese

12 ounces fat-free or low-fat plain Greek yogurt

2 whole eggs, whisked

2 egg whites

2 tablespoons agave nectar

2 scoops preferred protein powder

4 graham cracker sheets

2 tablespoons melted coconut oil

1 tablespoon unsweetened almond milk

1. Preheat oven to 250°F.

2. Let the cream cheese sit at room temperature to allow it to soften.

3. Mix together Greek yogurt, whole eggs, egg whites, agave nectar, and softened cream cheese in a medium bowl.

4. Add protein powder to the bowl, and mix well. Once mixed, set filling aside.

5. Crush up graham crackers until they resemble a powder. You can crush them by hand, but it is much easier to use a food processor if one is available.

6. Mix the crushed graham crackers with the coconut oil and the almond milk to form the crust.

7. Line an 8-inch round baking pan with parchment paper.

8. Flatten the crust into the baking pan using your hands. Try to make the crust lay as evenly as possible in the pan.

9. Pour the cheesecake filling into the crust. Spread the cheesecake mixture so it sits evenly throughout the pan.

10. Bake the cheesecake for 30 minutes at 250°F.

11. Lower the oven temperature to 220°F. Continue baking for another 40 minutes.

12. Remove the cheesecake from the oven and let cool on a baking rack for about 1 hour.

13. Once the cheesecake has cooled, place in the refrigerator for several hours to allow it to completely set.

Pumpkin Chocolate Cookies

MAKES: 12 cookies

COOK TIME: 35 minutes

2 scoops preferred vanilla protein powder

4 large egg whites

4 ounces pumpkin puree

1 (1/2-ounce) fat-free instant chocolate pudding mix

¼ teaspoon baking powder

¼ teaspoon vanilla extract

¼ teaspoon pumpkin spice blend

2 tablespoons stevia

¼ cup dark chocolate chips

coconut oil cooking spray

1. Preheat oven to 325°F.

2. Mix all ingredients except the coconut oil together in a large bowl, using a spatula or wooden spoon.

3. Spray baking sheet with coconut oil.

4. Spoon 12 scoops of dough onto baking sheet. Bake cookies at 325°F for 20 minutes or until golden brown.

5. Once cookies have cooled, refrigerate. Serve cookies chilled.

APPENDIX

GLOSSARY

Adiponectin. Adiponectin is a protein hormone that is secreted from fat cells. It helps regulate blood sugar levels and has a role in breaking down fatty acids. Adiponectin can affect how the body responds to insulin and can also have an anti-inflammatory effect on the blood vessels.

Adipose tissue. Adipose tissue is another name for body fat. The main purpose of fat is to store extra energy that our bodies don't need right away, but it also cushions and insulates our bodies. Depending on where you store your fat, it can be a greater health risk.

Aerobic exercise. Also known as cardio, aerobic exercise will get your heart rate up, and requires more oxygen. Examples of aerobic exercise include brisk walking, jogging, biking, and swimming.

Amino acids. Amino acids are considered the "building blocks" of protein. There are 20 different amino acids that make up our body proteins. Nine amino acids are considered essential, meaning that our bodies cannot make them, and they must come from the diet. Eleven amino acids are non-essential, meaning that our bodies can make them if we need them and are in short supply.

Blood glucose. Blood glucose, also referred to as blood sugar, means how much sugar is in your bloodstream at a certain time. We all need glucose to provide our cells with energy, but having high blood glucose can lead to a lot of health issues. Someone who is diabetic or pre-diabetic would likely have high blood glucose levels.

BMI. BMI is short for body mass index. To calculate BMI, you take your weight, in kilograms, and divide it by the square of your height, in meters ($BMI=Kg/m^2$). BMI is used to measure your body fat. Typically, a BMI under 18.5 is considered underweight, between 18.5 to 24.9 is considered normal, between 25 to 29.9 is considered overweight, and a BMI greater than 30 is considered obese.

Body composition. Body composition refers to what percentage of muscle, fat, bone, and water our bodies are made up of. The ideal body composition for each person is dependent on your biological sex, age, and fitness level.

Branched chain amino acids (BCAAs). Out of the 20 total amino acids, there are three branched chain amino acids. These are leucine, isoleucine, and valine. BCAAs are involved with protein synthesis, have roles in the immune system, and help with brain function. They are a popular choice among athletes, as they promote new muscle growth and may help reduce muscle breakdown during more intense exercises.

Cardiovascular disease. Cardiovascular disease, or heart disease, refers to a number of diseases that affect the heart and blood vessels. Some examples are coronary artery disease, high blood pressure (hypertension), or heart attack.

Complete protein. A protein is considered a complete protein if it contains all of the essential amino acids. Complete proteins usually come from animal foods, but some plant foods are considered complete proteins as well. Some examples of complete proteins are eggs, meat, poultry, fish, dairy products, whey protein, soy, amaranth, and quinoa.

Denaturing. This is the process by which proteins are exposed to some type of stress or heat that can cause them to start to break down, meaning that it will start to lose its shape and structure.

Ghrelin. Ghrelin is also known as the hunger hormone because it affects your appetite. When your stomach is empty, your body releases ghrelin to increase hunger. After you eat and your stomach is full, your body stops releasing ghrelin.

HDL cholesterol. HDL stands for high-density lipoprotein and is frequently referred to as the "good cholesterol." HDL cholesterol travels through the body and picks up LDL cholesterol, bringing it back to the liver to be processed.

Incomplete protein. A protein is considered an incomplete protein if it is missing one or more of the essential amino acids. Some plant-based foods are considered incomplete proteins. Examples of incomplete proteins include wheat, rice, peas, lentils, beans, nuts, and seeds. However, you can eat a combination of two incomplete proteins to create a complete protein food.

Insulin. Insulin is a hormone that is made by the pancreas. Although insulin has several functions, most people are familiar with insulin in relation to diabetes. One of insulin's jobs is to tell the cells in our bodies to take in glucose (sugar) from the blood-stream, which would lower the blood sugar level to a normal range. If someone is diabetic or pre-diabetic, they are either not making any insulin, not making enough insulin, or their cells are no longer responding to the insulin (see insulin resistance, below).

Insulin resistance. Insulin resistance is a condition in which someone's body stops responding to insulin the way that it should. Cells are resistant to the insulin and do not use insulin as well as they would in someone who does not have insulin resistance. This can lead to high blood sugar levels since their bodies' cells are not taking in glucose the way that they should. This can be a problem, as the pancreas will keep producing more insulin to try and return the blood sugar to a normal range. Eventually, the body will not be able to produce enough insulin to bring down blood sugars. Many people do not know that they are insulin resistant. Eventually, insulin resistance can turn into diabetes. Insulin resistance tends to be associated with being overweight or having a lot of visceral fat.

Insulin sensitivity. Insulin sensitivity means that you need only a small amount of insulin for your cells to take in a certain amount of glucose.

Interval training. Interval training is a type of exercise where you participate in very high intensity exercise followed by brief rest periods or lower intensity exercise. Interval training can be a very efficient way to improve your overall fitness level and burn body fat.

Glossary

Kilogram. A kilogram is equal to 2.2 pounds. I use a person's weight in kilograms to estimate calorie and protein needs. To determine your weight in kilograms, divide your total weight by 2.2. For example, someone who is 165 pounds is 75 kilograms (165 ÷ 2.2 = 75). In medical settings, dosages and calculations are almost always done based on your weight in kilograms.

LDL cholesterol. LDL stands for low-density lipoprotein. LDL cholesterol is also known as the "bad cholesterol." LDL cholesterol is considered bad because it can become part of the plaque that accumulates in the arteries of the heart, increasing your risk for developing heart disease.

Leptin. Leptin is another hormone that affects appetite and weight control. Leptin is produced by cells in the adipose tissue and helps regulate how much you are eating by stopping feelings of hunger. Leptin can be considered the opposite hormone of ghrelin. When someone is obese, they are not as sensitive to leptin, which can lead them to have a difficult time determining if they are full. Reduced sensitivity to leptin can lead to increased weight gain, which further decreases sensitivity, thereby worsening both conditions.

Lipids. When I am referring to blood lipid levels or a lipid panel, this is a type of lab test that is looking at the amount of fat in your blood. The different types of fats are the total blood cholesterol levels, triglyceride levels, HDL cholesterol levels, and LDL cholesterol levels. This is an important test to have done regularly to make sure that you are not at an increased risk for heart disease. High levels of cholesterol, triglycerides, and LDL cholesterol are a risk factor for heart disease.

Macronutrient. A macronutrient is something that we need to consume in large amounts for health and to sustain life. In human diets, the three major macronutrients are protein, carbohydrate, and fat. All three macronutrients have different roles and functions, but all can be used to provide energy. Overeating any of the macronutrients can lead to weight gain.

Metabolic syndrome. Metabolic syndrome is not a disease, but rather a set of problems that can lead you to develop heart disease and diabetes. These factors are high blood pressure, high fasting blood sugar, high triglyceride levels, low HDL cholesterol, and a large amount of visceral adipose tissue. You need at least three out of five factors for a diagnosis of metabolic syndrome. Losing weight is key to reversing metabolic syndrome and the potential poor health outcomes. Unfortunately, many people with metabolic syndrome have insulin resistance, which can make it more of a struggle to lose weight. This is why it is so important to try and lose weight if you are showing any of the risk factors for metabolic syndrome.

Metabolism. You may have heard people say that they have a fast metabolism or a slow metabolism. There are a number of things that can affect your metabolism, such as height and weight. A man who is 6 feet tall and 200 pounds needs a lot more calories than a man who is 5 feet tall and 120 pounds. The amount of muscle you have also affects your metabolism (more muscle = higher metabolism). Additionally, if a man and a woman are the same size, the man will usually have a higher metabolism, since men tend to have more muscle mass. Age also affects metabolism. As we get older, most people lose muscle mass and have more body fat, which slows down their metabolism. These things will affect your basal metabolic rate (the number of calories you normally burn during the day, even if you are resting).

Net protein utilization (NPU). Net protein utilization is another way of evaluating the overall quality of a protein. It refers to how usable a protein is. When a protein is digested, it is broken down into a certain number of amino acids. The amount of amino acids that are produced from a protein's breakdown after eating is compared to the amount of amino acids that are converted into a new protein. The higher the net protein utilization, the more effective the protein is.

PRISE. PRISE is a phrase that was used to describe a specific type of treatment given in protein pacing research studies. PRISE stands for protein pacing, resistance exercise, intervals, stretching/yoga/Pilates, and endurance exercise.

Protein digestibility. Protein digestibility is a way to evaluate protein quality by determining what proportion of the protein is absorbed by the body. While some products may have a higher protein content than others, they may be less digestible, which provides less benefit to the body.

Protein synthesis. Protein synthesis refers to how our bodies make and build new proteins from amino acids. Protein synthesis creates proteins for a number of reasons, from helping to make new parts of a cell to building new muscle.

Resting energy expenditure (REE). Resting energy expenditure refers to how many calories are required for your body to function over a 24-hour period when it is at rest.

Resistance training. Resistance training is a form of exercise that has your muscles showing resistance against a force. This is done to help improve the strength and size of different muscle groups. Regular resistance training can help you become stronger and improve bone density. By improving the strength and size of different muscle groups, resistance training can help increase metabolism.

Satellite cell. A satellite cell is a type of cell that exists in muscle tissue. When you participate in strength or resistance training, satellite cells will gather where there is damage to the muscle and help repair the injured area. Satellite cells will also fuse together leading to muscle gain, or muscle hypertrophy. Satellite cells are extremely important in muscle recovery and growth. Amino acids and protein intake are required for satellite cells to work properly.

Subcutaneous adipose tissue. Subcutaneous adipose tissue, or subcutaneous fat, is fat that is located just below the skin. Having excess subcutaneous adipose tissue is safer than having excess visceral adipose tissue, as this type of fat is not linked with an increased disease risk. Typically, people who have more subcutaneous adipose tissue than visceral adipose tissue are considered to be pear shaped.

Texturized vegetable protein (TVP). Texturized vegetable protein is a product that is made from soy flour. The proteins in soy flour are isolated and the resulting product, TVP, is often used as an alternative to meat. It can be used to make vegetarian burgers or hotdogs, and it adds well to many different types of recipes. It is an excellent protein option to add to your diet as it is a low-calorie and low-fat source of protein. Since it is derived from soy, it is also a complete protein.

Glossary

Thermic effect of food. The thermic effect of food refers to the increase in metabolism that happens after you eat a meal. Even though you consume calories when you eat, your body needs to use some energy (calories) to break down, absorb, and use the nutrients you have just eaten. The thermic effect of food is much higher for protein foods than it is for carbohydrates or fats (meaning that we burn a greater percentage of the calories trying to digest the protein foods). It also takes more calories to digest and absorb complex carbohydrates than it does simple, refined carbohydrates. It is estimated that we burn up to 5 percent of the total calories from dietary fat just from digestion; comparatively, we burn between 5 to 10 percent of the calories when we are eating carbohydrates, and 20 to 30 percent of the calories when we are eating protein foods.

Total cholesterol. Cholesterol is a fat-like material that is in all the cells of our body to help provide structure. Our bodies can make cholesterol, but it also is found in some foods that we eat. When people are said to have high cholesterol, they are referring to total cholesterol levels. While your body does require cholesterol to function, having too much cholesterol can increase the risk of heart disease. Total cholesterol means the total amount of all cholesterol in your blood, including both HDL and LDL cholesterol.

Triglycerides. Triglycerides are a type of fat in your blood that can become problematic at high levels. If they get too high, they can contribute to the development of heart disease.

Visceral adipose tissue. Visceral adipose tissue refers to the type of fat that is located around our internal organs. It is considered more dangerous than having fat located directly beneath our skin. Visceral adipose tissue is linked to an increased risk for heart disease, type II diabetes, and certain types of cancer. Visceral adipose tissue also produces hormones that can lead to health problems, including insulin resistance. People who have a lot of visceral adipose tissue are typically referred to as having an apple shape.

REFERENCES

While I was writing this book, I thought it was important that I be as accurate as possible, especially since this was an area that I had not practiced in yet. I ended up spending a lot of time doing research and looking up scientific articles in peer-reviewed journals. I would not have recommended any sort of program unless it was evidence-based and appropriate for someone to follow. The purpose of this book was to translate the research articles into simpler language that is easier to understand and follow. I also wanted to give credit to the original study authors. However, if you have any interest in reading the original articles or educating yourself further, I have included all my references.

Arciero, Paul J., Daniel Baur, et al. "Timed-Daily Ingestion of Whey Protein and Exercise Training Reduces Visceral Adipose Tissue Mass and Improves Insulin Resistance: the PRISE Study." *Journal of Applied Physiology* 117, no. 1 (2014):1–10. doi:10.1152/japplphysiol.00152.2014.

Arciero, Paul J., Rohan C. Edmonds, et al. "Protein Pacing from Food or Supplementation Improves Physical Performance in Overweight Men and Women: The PRISE 2 Study." *Nutrients* 8, no. 5 (2016):288. doi:10.3390/nu8050288.

Arciero, Paul J., Rohan Edmonds, et al. "Protein Pacing Caloric-Restriction Enhances Body Composition Similarly in Obese Men and Women During Weight Loss and Sustains Efficacy During Long-Term Weight Maintenance." *Nutrients* 8, no. 8 (2016):476. doi:10.3390/nu8080476.

Arciero, Paul J., Stephen J. Ives, et al. "Protein Pacing and Multi-Component Exercise Training Improves Physical Performance Outcomes in Exercise-Trained Women: The PRISE 3 Study." *Nutrients* 8 no. 6 (2016):332. doi:10.3390/nu8060332.

Baer, David J., Kim S. Stote, et al. "Whey Protein but Not Soy Protein Supplementation Alters Body Weight and Composition in Free-Living Overweight and Obese Adults." *The Journal of Nutrition* 141, no 8 (2011):1489–1494. doi:10.3945/jn.111.139840.

Garaulet, Marta, Purificación Gómez-Abellán, et al. "Timing of Food Intake Predicts Weight Loss Effectiveness." *International Journal of Obesity* 37, no 4 (2013):604–611. doi:10.1038/ijo.2013.18.

Giezenaar, Caroline, Zoé Coudert, et al. "Effects of Timing of Whey Protein Intake on Appetite and Energy Intake in Healthy Older Men." *Journal of the American Medical Directors Association* 18, no 10 (2017). doi:10.1016/j.jamda.2017.06.027.

Hoffman, Jay R. "Protein Intake: Effect of Timing." *Strength and Conditioning Journal* 29, no. 6 (2007):26. doi:10.1519/00126548-200712000-00005.

References

Ives, Stephen, Chelsea Norton, et al. "Multi-Modal Exercise Training and Protein Pacing Enhances Physical Performance Adaptations Independent of Growth Hormone and BDNF but May Be Dependent on IGF-1 in Exercise-Trained Men." *Growth Hormone & IGF Research* 32 (2017):60–70. doi:10.1016/j.ghir.2016.10.002.

Jäger, Ralf, Chad M. Kerksick, et al. "International Society of Sports Nutrition Position Stand: Protein and Exercise." *Journal of the International Society of Sports Nutrition* 14, no. 20 (2017). doi:10.1186/s12970-017-0177-8.

Mirtschink, Peter, Cholsoon Jang, et al. "Fructose Metabolism, Cardiometabolic Risk, and the Epidemic of Coronary Artery Disease." *European Heart Journal* (2017). doi:10.1093/eurheartj/ehx518.

INDEX

Index

Index

Recipe Contributors

While I have been a registered dietitian for nearly 10 years, recipe development has never been my strong suit. So I collaborated with New Leaf Fitness & Nutrition on some recipes. I cannot express how much gratitude I have for their assistance. These recipes are courtesy of New Leaf: Purple People Eater Smoothie, EspressPro Smoothie, Monkey's Lunch Smoothie, Protein Acai-Fruit Bowl, Peanut Butter and Jelly Ice Cream Smoothie, Strawberry Banana High-Protein Shake, Banana Oatmeal Protein Muffins, Fat-Free Pumpkin Pancakes, Low-Carb Pancakes, Two-Ingredient Banana Pancakes, High-Protein Overnight Oats, Apple Cinnamon Overnight Oats, and Protein Pudding.

New Leaf Fitness & Nutrition (www.newleaffitness.org) takes a positive holistic approach to fitness and nutrition. It's not just about looking good; it's about feeling good, too. It isn't about losing weight or gaining muscle; It's about finding a balance that's right for you and your lifestyle, progressing each day to develop yourself physically and mentally, as well.

New Leaf's programs are designed with three things in mind: health, goals, and balance. They offer meal plans that vary from selected dieting, flexible meal planning, or macro counting, all the while taking into consideration the client's likes, dislikes, and limitations. Programs are designed specifically for you and your lifestyle, to help reach your goals with the tools to live a balanced life and improve your personal fitness, health, mental health, energy, and positive attitude toward fitness and food. Find New Leaf on Instagram @newleaffitness and #newleafit.